Young People, Social Media and Health

The pervasiveness of social media in young people's lives is widely acknow-ledged, yet there is little evidence-based understanding of the impacts of social media on young people's health and wellbeing.

Young People, Social Media and Health draws on novel research to under-stand, explain, and illustrate young people's experiences of engagement with health-related social media; as well as the impacts they report on their health, wellbeing, and physical activity. Using empirical case studies, digital representa-tions, and evidence from multi-sector and interdisciplinary stakeholders and aca-demics, this volume identifies the opportunities and risk-related impacts of social media.

Offering new theoretical insights and practical guidelines for educators, prac-titioners, parents/guardians, and policy makers; *Young People, Social Media and Health* will also appeal to students and researchers interested in fields such as Sociology of Sport, Youth Sports Development, Secondary Physical Education, and Media Effects.

Victoria A. Goodyear is a Lecturer in Pedagogy in the School of Sport, Exer-cise and Rehabilitation Sciences, University of Birmingham, UK.

Kathleen M. Armour is Pro-Vice-Chancellor (Education) and the academic lead for the Higher Education Futures institute (HEFi), University of Birmingham, UK.

Routledge Studies in Physical Education and Youth Sport
Series Editor: David Kirk
University of Strathclyde, UK

The *Routledge Studies in Physical Education and Youth Sport* series is a forum for the discussion of the latest and most important ideas and issues in physical education, sport, and active leisure for young people across school, club, and recreational settings. The series presents the work of the best well-established and emerging scholars from around the world, offering a truly international perspective on policy and practice. It aims to enhance our understanding of key challenges, to inform academic debate, and to have a high impact on both policy and practice, and is thus an essential resource for all serious students of physical education and youth sport.

Also available in this series

www.routledge.com/sport/series/RSPEYS

Young People, Social Media and Health

Edited by Victoria A. Goodyear and
Kathleen M. Armour

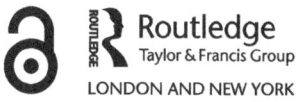

LONDON AND NEW YORK

First published 2019
by Routledge
2 Park Square, Milton Park, Abingdon, Oxon OX14 4RN

and by Routledge
52 Vanderbilt Avenue, New York, NY 10017, USA

First issued in paperback 2020

Routledge is an imprint of the Taylor & Francis Group, an informa business

British Library Cataloguing-in-Publication Data
A catalogue record for this book is available from the British Library

Library of Congress Cataloging-in-Publication Data
Names: Goodyear, Victoria A., author. | Armour, Kathleen M., author.
Title: Young people, social media and health / Victoria A. Goodyear and
Kathleen M. Armour.
Description: Abingdon, Oxon ; New York, NY : Routledge, 2018. | Series:
Routledge studies in physical education and youth sport | Includes
bibliographical references and index.
Identifiers: LCCN 2018035743| ISBN 9781138493957 (hardback) |
ISBN 9781351026987 (ebk)
Subjects: LCSH: Social media in medicine. | Internet and teenagers.
Classification: LCC R859.7.S63 G66 2018 | DDC 610.2850835–dc23
LC record available at https://lccn.loc.gov/2018035743

ISBN 13: 978-0-367-66467-1 (pbk)
ISBN 13: 978-1-138-49395-7 (hbk)

Typeset in Times New Roman
by Wearset Ltd, Boldon, Tyne and Wear

Contents

17 Young people, social media, physical activity, and health: final thoughts on the work, the present, and the future   212

LORRAINE CALE

Figures

Tables

Contributors

Kathleen M. Armour, Pro-Vice-Chancellor Education, University of Birmingham, UK.

Penny Van Bergen, Centre for Children's Learning in a Social World, Macquarie University, Australia.

Lorraine Cale, School of Sport, Exercise and Health Sciences, Loughborough University, UK.

Ashley Casey, School of Sport, Exercise and Health Sciences, Loughborough University, UK.

Dean A. Dudley, Centre for Children's Learning in a Social World, Department of Educational Studies, Macquarie University, Australia.

Eimear Enright, School of Human Movement and Nutrition Sciences, University of Queensland, Australia.

Michael Gard, School of Human Movement and Nutrition Sciences, University of Queensland, Australia.

Victoria A. Goodyear, School of Sport, Exercise and Rehabilitation Sciences, University of Birmingham, UK.

David Kirk, School of Education, Strathclyde University, UK and School of Human Movement and Nutrition Sciences, University of Queensland, Australia.

Erin Mackenzie, Centre for Children's Learning in a Social World, Macquarie University, Australia.

Anne McMaugh, Centre for Children's Learning in a Social World, Macquarie University, Australia.

Anthony Papathomas, School of Sport, Exercise and Health Sciences, Loughborough University, UK.

Carolyn R. Plateau, School of Sport, Exercise and Health Sciences, Loughborough University, UK.

Thomas Quarmby, Carnegie School of Sport, Leeds Beckett University, UK.

Mikael Quennerstedt, School of Health Sciences, Örebro University, Sweden.

Emma Rich, Department for Health, Bath University, UK.

Rachel Sandford, School of Sport, Exercise and Health Sciences, Loughborough University, UK.

Brett Smith, School of Sport, Exercise and Rehabilitation Sciences, University of Birmingham, UK.

Hannah J. White, School of Sport, Exercise and Health Sciences, Loughborough University, UK.

Hannah Wood, School of Sport, Exercise and Rehabilitation Sciences, University of Birmingham, UK.

Foreword

Brett Smith

I'm an academic who seeks to critically examine health, promote good qualitative inquiry, engage in research co-production, and think with stories and theory. I also dabble with certain social media, like Twitter. But I am much more than an academic; I am father too.

As a 'Daddy' of a young son who is at school I feel compelled to better understand social media as an important space and place in which humans and the material intra-act, how we are influenced and influencing. When I think of my young boy and his possible futures in terms of social media, I am excited, delighted, thrilled, worried, troubled, angry, frustrated, confused, and perplexed; emotions and feelings spill out. I sometimes wonder how other parents, as well as teachers, might feel about social media? What do they do? How can we become more aware of the opportunities and risk-related impacts of social media on young people's health? How might we support and work with young people across the life course to engage with health-related social media in positive ways? How might we – parents, teachers, and various stakeholders – negotiate the tethering of young people to social media and productively navigate the complex process of different bodies acting and becoming with ever-increasing new material realities? And, of course, what about young people themselves? What do they think and feel? How do they act on and with social media? How do social media act on, in, and with young people, and with what affects? What harmful and beneficial impacts do social media have on their health and wellbeing? How to they navigate a complex digital world, and what might be at stake for their health, wellbeing, and our futures?

Rather uniquely, this book eloquently offers responses to such questions – and foregrounds and provokes many more. A book like this is therefore welcomed. It builds on and significantly extends recent calls to take young people, social media, digital technology, physical activity, and health seriously. The editors and chapter contributors are experts in the cases and topics they present. Each offers valuable insights and messages into contemporary issues that are timely for many people, groups, and organisations. The book breaks new ground by bringing together a collection of esteemed authors, methods, methodologies, epistemologies, ontologies, and theories that illuminate and explain important issues for societies. I expect it will become an invaluable resource for novice and experienced researchers alike. It is hoped too that the book will reach audiences beyond those across academia and be meaningful for them. This hope might be realised when one considers such matters as narrative, communication, knowledge translation, qualitative research, and co-production.

This book first offers six evidence-based composite narrative case studies. These were constructed from the editors' funded research projects undertaken *with* over 1,346 young people from the UK – a point I will return to. But first the value of narrative needs highlighting. Narratives are popular forms of data for researchers to analyse. Our analysis of stories can provide valuable insights into people's meaning-making, experiences, materiality, and sociocultural worlds. Stories can also function as highly effective forms of communication. They can communicate complex knowledge in ways that are highly accessible to different audiences, not just academics. There are many reasons for this. Stories can have the capacity to attract people, hold their attention, and get under their skin. Memory is partly story-based, and, as a consequence, knowledge can be 'absorbed', 'integrated', and 'remembered' through stories. Stories further can generate emotional impact. They have the capacity to make things not only plausible but also compelling. They can resonate, allow different perspectives to be imagined, elicit feelings, and make life dramatic. In doing so, stories have the additional capacity to then act on us, arousing emotions, affecting how we think, feel, and might behave. That is, stories can do crucial things to, with, in, and on us.

It is no accident then that the editors gave stories a central stage to act via this book. Of course, stories are always out of control. We cannot predict what they do on people or how people might engage with them. But by ensuring stories are a key part of the book, and bringing each story together in it, the chances that the research will be communicated to people beyond academia is significantly enhanced. With the editors, I hope then the stories do various things. That includes communicating vital knowledge so that awareness of the opportunities and risk-related impacts of social media on young people's health are expanded. In such ways, the stories in the book can be viewed and used as a form of 'knowledge tool' – a focused and evidence-based resource that disseminates knowledge to potentially large audiences.

The stories however were not taken from young people and then turned into a tale the authors wanted to spin only by themselves. What is important is that the research in the book was conducted with young people, not on them. From the beginning, the team co-produced the research the book showcases. For instance, young people and key stakeholders (e.g. schools, teachers, physical activity and health leaders in community settings, and policy and industry professionals) spent much time creating research questions, analysing data, questioning the researchers, and thinking through complex issues about social media, health, and wellbeing that the stories seek to show. The book thus supports and adds to calls for more qualitative research that is participatory. It also pushes qualitative researchers to think about how digital media can be harnessed as not only a 'method' for collecting data and understanding people and groups. The book raises questions about the post-digital, how we might enact research differently for different purposes, and how we might communicate research beyond the textual, for example.

The stories that form part of the book are useful as standalone resources for communicating research, engaging different readers, and thinking about qualitative research. It is however also pleasing to see part of the book devoted to engaging in theorising. The book showcases differing theories about young people, social media, digital technology, physical activity, and health. The chapter contributors do not seek to offer the last word – finalise – about the stories presented early in the book. They leave the readers with the view that stories and lives can and do change, leaving people unfinalised. The chapter contributors likewise theorise the stories that form the first part of book with care, sophistication, and an openness for other theoretical possibilities. On the one hand, they bring theory to life by connecting it to stories. On the other hand, they put stories to scholarly work by engaging with them theoretically. It is refreshing to see a book that delivers an eclectic range of theorising into young people's digital health and related behaviours.

I hope readers will appreciate the book as much as I did. Like concentric circles of witness, it is hoped that book teaches, reaches different audiences, makes a difference, and opens up possible new worlds. Enjoy!

Preface

Thank you, to the young people involved in the underpinning research of this book, for their time, enthusiasm, and willingness to share their experiences. We are also indebted to their schools and teachers, who facilitated the ability to work with the young people, and JustJag for helping us to communicate young people's stories through the medium of digital animated videos.

We would also like to thank the key stakeholders involved in the research and the chapter authors of this book, for their important, significant, and critical insights. We are also grateful to the Wellcome Trust for funding this research and ensuring that this book is open access and can reach the widest possible audience.

1 What young people tell us about health-related social media and why we should listen

Victoria A. Goodyear and Kathleen M. Armour

Chapter overview

The pervasiveness of social media in young people's lives is widely acknowledged; yet, there is little robust evidence on the impacts of social media on young people's health and wellbeing. In this chapter, we explain the innovative research we have undertaken to understand, from young people's perspectives, the health-related issues and opportunities of social media. We explain key terms, including the new 'content-led pedagogical framework' and the 'pedagogical case model'. These tools were used to present, analyse, explain, and translate empirically rich data on young people's experiences of social media, and from stakeholder and academic groups from a range of disciplines.

The focus of the book

For many of the young people that we teach, coach, research, care for, parent, and support, it is important to remember that digital technology is regarded as an extension of self and social media is a primary mode of communication and social engagement. If, as adults, we want to reach these young people, understand something of their worlds, and offer support, we need to know how they engage with social media, what they learn from it and how that may influence their behaviours (Goodyear *et al.* 2018a, 2018b). While many influences may be positive, there are also likely to be periods of vulnerability in young people's lives where the sheer scale, intensity, and pervasiveness of social media could act to intensify those vulnerabilities. Social media is certainly a very powerful and dynamic feature of contemporary youth culture and, as such, it is important to understand how it operates in key areas of young people's lives.

This book adopts a novel approach to understanding, explaining, and communicating young people's experiences of health-related social media, and the impacts they report on their health, wellbeing, and levels of physical activity. The chapters are underpinned by robust data. Using empirically rich composite narrative case studies and evidence from multi-sector and multi-disciplinary stakeholders and academics, the book identifies the opportunities and risk-related impacts of social media for young people's health and wellbeing. It offers new theoretical insights, as well as evidence-based and practical guidelines for relevant stakeholders including policy makers, schools, and health and education professionals/practitioners. The evidence presented in this book also provides information that will be important for parents/guardians and will help them to better understand how to engage with and respond to young people's contemporary needs.

The significance of this book resides in the insights it offers to address growing concerns around the world about young people's health and wellbeing (Inchley *et al.* 2017; Patton *et al.* 2016), and reported associations between young people's uses of social media and negative physical and mental health outcomes (Frith 2017; Swist *et al.* 2015; Third *et al.* 2017). Yet, there is limited robust evidence that explains whether and how social media influences young people's health-related knowledge and behaviours (Przybylski and Weinstein 2017a, 2017b). As a result, many adults are uncertain about how to support young people's engagement with health-related social media (Shaw *et al.* 2015; Third *et al.* 2017) and there is little guidance available from research and policy (Third *et al.* 2017; Wartella *et al.* 2016). This leaves adults ill-equipped both to protect young people from the negative influences of social media and to optimise the potential of social media as a medium for health promotion. This book, therefore, addresses a persistent societal question in new ways, and provides important evidence-based insights that are relevant to policy makers, researchers, health and education practitioners/professionals, and parents/guardians who have an interest in supporting young people's health-related understandings and behaviours.

The book is organised into three main parts, and each can be read independently or in any order. In Part I, a series of data-rich case studies illustrates some of the many ways in which young people engage with social media and how and why this can have an influence on their health-related knowledge, understandings, and behaviours. In Part II, we step back from the vivid data and draw on a range of different disciplinary perspectives to better understand the ways in which health-related social media can influence young people. In Part III, the information from the previous sections is crystallised into evidence-based actions and guidelines that can help relevant adults to mitigate against risks while simultaneously maximising the positive and powerful potential of engagement with digital health-related media.

The importance of new research on social media that listens to young people

It has been reported from numerous international and socio-economic contexts that young people have the highest rates of social media use of any age group, and that they spend significant proportions of their time 'on' social media (Royal Society of Public Health [RPSH] 2017; Third *et al.* 2017). Turkle (2017) used the concept of 'tethered' to describe young people's prolific uses of social media and to highlight that young people want to be continuously 'connected'. Others have argued that young people's extensive and habitual uses of social media challenge the outdated notion that a dualism exists between 'real' life and online spaces (boyd 2014; Ito *et al.* 2010; Third *et al.* 2014). A dissolution of the online/offline binary is made apparent where social media operates as an active digital space for young people where relationships, identities, and intimacies are formed (boyd 2014; Handyside and Ringrose 2017; MacIsaac *et al.* 2018), and where learning can occur as a result of observing and communicating with peers of the same age (Ito *et al.* 2010). In this sense, social media is not merely a space where young people go to document their lives (Handyside and Ringrose 2017). Social media is a connected space for young people where communication, friendship, play, self-expression, and learning occur (Handyside and Ringrose 2017, MacIsaac *et al.* 2018).

There can be little doubt that understanding how social media influences young people's knowledge and behaviour is highly complex and difficult to navigate. There are diverse modes of social media (e.g. Snapchat or Instagram) that include varied and multi-dimensional interactive functionalities (e.g. likes or followers) (Highfield and Leaver 2016). The content created and accessed on social media is also user-generated, and shared in spaces where commercial, government, community, and individual contexts overlap (Freishtat and Sandlin 2010). In turn, social media disrupts the flow of traditional forms of health knowledge, where established learning and pedagogical concepts, procedures, and frameworks are problematic to apply in this highly interactive and dynamic context (Andersson and Öhman 2017; Andersson and Olson 2014; Goodyear 2017; Goodyear *et al.* 2018a). Understanding how social media influences knowledge and behaviour is even more challenging given that this medium is in a constant flux of change. New platforms, functions, and features are frequently introduced and adopted in youth culture (Miller *et al.* 2016), such as the rapid uptake of Snapchat in recent years that has, in turn, presented new issues related to temporality and memory (Handyside and Ringrose 2017; Highfield and Leaver 2016). Social media is, therefore, a very contemporary, dynamic, and interactive medium that engages young people. Navigating this type of media and understanding how the diverse, multi-user, and multi-functional spaces influence young people's knowledge and understanding is methodologically, theoretically, and ethically challenging.

To date, understandings of the health-related risks and opportunities of social media have been undermined by methodological weakness (Gaplin and Taylor 2017). Most studies fail to reflect the social complexity of the medium and/or the diverse ways in which young people navigate it. Evidence has been limited to one-off, short-duration intervention studies, analysis of parent/guardian and teacher perspectives, and/or evidence from survey data or observational methods (James 2014; Mascheroni, Jorge, and Farrugia 2014; Wartella *et al.* 2016). From these studies, health-related impacts of digital media engagement have been associated with time spent on social media, the platform, and/or the dissemination/accessibility of information (RPSH 2017; Shaw *et al.* 2015). Yet, the dynamic ways in which young people interact through social media (see boyd

2014), and the powerful role of, for example, peers (Ito *et al.* 2010), likes (Jong and Drummond 2016), followers (MacIsaac *et al.* 2018), and selfies (Walsh 2017) are rarely considered. To understand how social media influences knowledge and behaviours, research must therefore account for the diverse multi-user and multi-functional interactive spaces of social media, and seek to better understand how young people use, navigate, and orientate themselves to these spaces.

The pressing need for new evidence on the dynamic and interactive ways in which young people engage with health-related social media is further indicated by the clear gaps that exist between adults and young people's understandings, where these gaps have been persistent (Buckingham 2016). International evidence suggests that young people value the accessibility of information from social media, and that they are increasingly turning to social media for health-related information (Swist *et al.* 2015; Third *et al.* 2017; Wartella *et al.* 2016). In existing research, young people have also reported on the benefits of social media in areas ranging from learning, socialisation, greater levels of social and emotional support, and creativity (Frith 2017; Swist *et al.* 2015; Third *et al.* 2017). Public discourse, however, tends to almost exclusively focus on social media and risk (boyd 2014). Adults also tend to assume that access to health information through social media will have negative knowledge-transmission effects that will impact on all young people in the same way (Third *et al.* 2017, 2014). Due to these perceived risks, there is a tendency to adopt protection-orientated approaches that seek to limit and control young people's social media use (boyd 2014; Livingstone, Mascheroni, and Staksrud 2018). As a result, many adults are unaware of the potential for social media to act as a positive health promotion resource and they fail to appreciate the opportunities that could stem from the dynamic and interactive ways in which young people use and navigate social media.

Despite young people's prolific engagement with social media, we, like others (Buckingham 2016; Hopkins 2010), are cautious of referring to the current generation as digital 'natives' or a digital youth generation. Nonetheless, we suggest that young people's very specific levels and forms of expertise in social media use should be recognised and accommodated. It is clear that young people are avid users and drivers of this contemporary, participatory, and user-driven online culture and, to this extent, they can be understood as highly skilled and knowledgeable. Understanding the ways in which young people use social media as a space for communication, entertainment, and learning could certainly challenge the social and cultural norms and expectations of adults (Ito *et al.* 2010; Livingstone *et al.* 2018). In the context of physical activity and health, for example, it has long been argued that understanding young people's perspectives is a powerful mechanism for designing new and more effective health and education interventions (Oliver and Kirk 2016; Leahy *et al.* 2016).

To understand how to better support young people's engagement with health-related social media, we argue that there is a need to learn from the experiences of young people. Any new guidelines or proposed interventions must chime with young people's needs and the ways in which they engage with social media. Developmentally, we know that adolescence is characterised by dynamic brain development and that interaction with the social environment shapes the capabilities an individual takes forward into adult life (Patton *et al.* 2016). In this context, social media can be a powerful social environment that can influence young people's current and future health-related behaviours. We also know that during adolescence, young people's social, emotional, and physical needs can change very rapidly, and this reinforces the need for relevant adults to be better informed about social media in order to offer appropriate support at particular points in time when young people might suddenly become vulnerable.

This book, therefore, addresses empirical, methodological, and theoretical gaps in our understandings about young people's engagement with health-related social media, and identifies new directions for research, policy, and practice. The aims of the book are to: (i) increase awareness of the opportunities and risk-related impacts of social media on young people's health; (ii) generate new theoretical insights into young people's digital health and related behaviours; and (iii) inform new guidelines and actions for health and education practitioners and other relevant adults who have a role in supporting young people to engage with health-related social media in positive ways. In this chapter, we set the context for the book by: (1) providing an overview of the underpinning research project that generated the data for the case study chapters; (2) reviewing existing research and theory in the area of social media and young people; (3) proposing a refined understanding of the concept of pedagogy to better account for the findings from our research and that of others; and (4) providing a guide to the structure and organisation of the book and each chapter.

New research: how we generated the data for the case study chapters

The underpinning research for this book was undertaken at the University of Birmingham (UK) and was supported by the Wellcome Trust.[1] Focusing on the key content areas of physical activity, diet/nutrition, and body image, we – Goodyear and Armour – sought to better understand from young people's perspectives, the health-related opportunities and issues generated by social media engagement. Between 2016–2017 we worked with a total of 1,346 young people and 35 key stakeholders working in areas related to young people's health and wellbeing. The project took place in three overarching phases.

Phase one of the research involved data collection in schools with young people. The aim was to generate new evidence on the types of health-related content young people access from social media, and to identify the types of content that they report as having an impact on their health-related knowledge and behaviours. Data collection involved 1,296 young people (age 13–18) from ten UK schools. The schools were located in diverse socio-demographic areas and the research included students from a range of ethnic backgrounds. A culturally responsive relational and reflexive approach to ethics was adopted (Sparkes and Smith 2014). This approach meant that ethical decision-making was guided by young people's needs and an awareness, understanding, and respect for their digital cultures (Goodyear 2017). Following this approach, data collection methods ensured participant safety, privacy, dignity, and autonomy. Informed consent and assent were provided, and legal conditions of social media were followed. Ethical approval was provided by The University of Birmingham Ethical Committee in July 2016.

In phase one, the data collection methods were initially co-constructed and then piloted with a group of ten young people (age 16–18), to ensure that the young people were able to communicate their experiences of social media. Participatory activities then took place in 12 different classes of young people across the ten schools ($n=236$, age 13–15, m$=101$, f$=135$). The class activities involved the young people working in small groups to complete a series of tasks on an iBook and included: watching a video, completing a leaflet, and editing and creating a Pinterest digital pinboard. Using the data generated from the class activities, 19 focus group interviews ($n=84$, age 13–15, m$=35$, f$=49$) took place with groups of young people from the class activities. Based on the data generated from the class activities and the interviews, an online survey was designed to 'test' the data in a wider sample of 1,016 young people within the same ten schools (age 13–16, m$=334$, f$=676$). The data from class activities, interviews, and the survey were then analysed using an adapted public pedagogies framework (explained in further detail below). The five themes that were constructed from the analysis process are reported in Chapters 2–7 and in the form of case study narratives. Further details on the methods and the analysis process can be found in Goodyear *et al.* (2018a).

Phase two of the research comprised of a workshop with 35 key stakeholders who have a responsibility for young people's health and wellbeing. The aim was to develop new guidelines and actions to help policy makers, researchers, health and education practitioners/professionals, and parents/guardians to support young people's engagement with health-related social media. Prior to the workshop, the text-based case studies (Chapters 2–7) were developed into short, 2–3-minute digital animated case study videos. Grounded in the knowledge-to-action knowledge translation framework (Graham *et al.* 2006) the videos were created as knowledge translation tools to: (i) present the case study data in a clear, concise, user-friendly, and accessible format; and (ii) help stakeholders to identify, select, and create appropriate guidance and actions. The data-rich videos can be accessed here:

http://epapers.bham.ac.uk/view/subjects/RC1200.html#group_G

The videos were presented to the stakeholders during the workshop and they were asked to provide an analysis of the risks and opportunities from their perspectives and to identify key actions. The profile of the stakeholder group was international, multi-sector, and multi-disciplinary and included teachers, international academics (UK, Ireland, Sweden, Netherlands, Spain, Australia, China), and trusts/organisations in the UK (such as the National Health service (NHS), Youth Sport Trust) that have a focus on youth health and wellbeing. The diversity of this stakeholder group resulted in insights into the case study data that were invaluable in seeking to reflect the diverse needs of young people and relevant adults. The stakeholder responses to the digital animated case study videos are reported in Chapters 2–7. In Chapters 8–15, a further theoretical analysis of the case studies is provided by some of the stakeholders who attended the workshop.

Phase three involved a workshop with 50 young people (age 13–16) from the ten schools that were involved in the data collection activities during phase one. Further grounded in the knowledge-to-action knowledge translation framework (Graham *et al.* 2006), the aims of this phase were to: (i) understand from the perspective of young people whether the guidelines and actions created by the stakeholders (phase two) were appropriate and would be effective; and (ii) identify the forms of support that young people perceive they require from adults. During the workshop, the young people watched the digital animated case study videos (phase two) and were presented with the responses of the stakeholders. In small groups, the young people then created a response for adults using artefacts explaining how young people their age should be supported to use social media for their health and wellbeing. The young people created and presented their response in different formats: radio or TV interviews, podcasts, movies, and newspaper articles. The data from the workshop were transcribed and then analysed using inductive and comparative techniques. The findings on how young people perceive adults should provide support is reported in Chapter 7. In the final step of the research, the data generated from the stakeholder (phase two) and young people (phase three) workshops were combined and further analysed. This analysis resulted in the development of evidence-based guidelines and actions that take into account stakeholder and young people's perspectives. These guidelines and actions can be accessed from Goodyear *et al.* (2018b).

The multi-layered, co-constructed, and participatory methods that were used in the project that underpins this book have ensured that the chapters are data-rich and evidence-based. In the next section, we summarise the broader evidence-base in which the project is located. This provided the grounding for our focus on listening to young people, and the methodological and conceptual approaches that we adopted.

Existing research: what can we learn from a review of the research on young people and social media

Pioneering work in the study of young people and social media has been undertaken mainly in the fields of anthropology, psychology, and sociology. The research in these disciplines has provided important insights into the opportunities presented by social media. Research led, for example, by boyd, Ito, Livingstone, James, and Ringrose has identified opportunities for informal learning, identify formation, media/digital literacy, and understanding ethics and feminism/gender. This research provides an appropriate foundation for understanding how social media might influence young people's health-related knowledge and behaviours, and identifying risks and opportunities, as well as theoretical and conceptual orientations that might develop new understandings.

boyd (2014, 2007) is a notable pioneer in defining and characterising young people's participation in social media. Grounded in anthropology, boyd (2007) used the concept of networked publics to describe how young people's participation in social media is interconnected to the notion of an audience. boyd (2014, p. 8) argued that networked publics are: 'simultaneously (1) the space constructed through networked technologies and (2) the imagined community that emerges as a result of the intersection of people, technology and practice'. boyd (2014, 2007) claimed that networked publics have four main affordances that alter and amplify social dynamics: persistence, visibility, spreadability, and searchability (boyd 2014, 2007). While these affordances present new opportunities for young people's development by extending their capabilities to engage with established practices – such as socialisation, self-expression, and the sharing of information – many young people use social media to attract attention and increase visibility (boyd 2014). Although some adults find this behaviour concerning and even alarming, boyd (2014) argued that these 'teen' behaviours on social media are no different to those of a pre-digital age. As a result, boyd (2014) argued that networked publics are significant to the needs of young people and, for some, offer a lifeline to engage in socialisation activities (boyd 2014).

Similar to boyd (2007), Ito *et al.* (2010, p. 19) used the term networked publics to 'foreground the active participation of a distributed social network in the production and circulation of culture and knowledge'. In their anthropological work with young people, Ito *et al.* (2010) noted that networked publics created a powerful context for peer-based learning and they proposed that learning occurs in two types of networked publics: friendship-driven and interest-driven. Friendship-driven publics are spaces for social and emotional support, where young people engage in self-expression and both evaluate and give feedback to one another. Interest-driven publics are more specialised and niche, and are centred on a common topic. Interest-driven publics influence learning through young people's interactions with others who have greater expertise and/ or where young people can mentor others while simultaneously developing their leadership skills. The work of Ito *et al.* (2010), therefore, suggests that young people's health-related learning could be enhanced through the increased opportunities for socialisation that are provided by social media and through peer-based and interest-driven networks.

The importance of digital media for young people's learning, wellbeing and socialisation is reflected in the extensive body of work led by Livingstone (see Livingstone *et al.* 2018). From a social psychology perspective, Livingstone has explored how the changing conditions of mediation reshape everyday practices and present new risks and opportunities for young people's wellbeing. In terms of risks, Livingstone reported that young people are exposed to a significant amount of harmful, user-generated content, including in the areas of health. Examples include pro-anorexic or self-harm content (Livingstone *et al.* 2014).

Yet, Livingstone *et al.* (2018) also reported that the risks for internet-using-young people are relatively low and exposure to content does not necessarily lead to harm. Based on these understandings, Livingstone, as well as others (see Third *et al.* 2014, 2017), have argued for digital access to be conceptualised as a fundamental 'right' for young people (Livingstone and Third 2017). From this rights-based perspective, Livingstone *et al.* (2018) called for a focus on media literacy which involves empowering young people to engage with society through the media. By engaging with the media, Livingstone (2017) argues that young people will develop the skills and knowledge they need to engage effectively with social media, and the skills to determine what information is useful, misleading, trusted, and/or stems from political or commercial interests (Livingstone 2017). Fundamental to Livingstone's (2017) argument is that the more media literacy skills young people gain, the more opportunities they will be afforded.

While the works of boyd, Ito *et al.* and Livingstone suggest that that social media engagement can lead to positive impacts on young people's health-related knowledge and behaviours, there are a number of more pessimistic viewpoints. Turkle (2017), for example, has outlined troubling consequences related to attention, thinking, identities, and relationships. In particular, Turkle (2017) claimed that young people's addiction to social media can result in social alienation, hinder the ability to engage in interpersonal communications, and lead to the development of shallow relationships focused on self-expression. This view is further supported by Gardner and Davis (2014), who argued that young people's dependency on social media apps could undermine the development of healthy identities and relationships, and the capacity to think creatively.

The work of James and colleagues highlights the potentially problematic moral and ethical consequences resulting from young people's engagement with digital media (James 2014; James *et al.* 2014). Drawing on psychological models of moral development (see James *et al.*, 2014), James (2014) outlined three ways in which young people approach digital media: self-focused, that involves a young person engaging with online activities where they mainly think about themselves; moral-focused, where a young person considers the consequences of online behaviour for other people they know; and ethically focused, where a young person considers the consequences of their behaviour for unknown individuals in wider social networks. The problematic issue for James (2014, p. 7) was that young people were 'principally, if not exclusively, concerned with their own interests when making decisions online'. This self-focused behaviour was reported, in some cases, to result in harm to a young person's peers and/or other individuals who were unknown to the young person. In this sense, while Livingstone (2017) suggests that media literacy will support young people's capacity to think critically about the digital information they encounter, James' (2014) research concludes that young people's understanding about how their individual behaviour impacts on others should also be addressed.

The importance of understanding how young people behave in their engagement with social media is further reflected in the research on gender and sexuality. Similar to James (2014), a number of scholars have pointed out that self-presentation on social media is of central importance to young people, and can drive the ways in which they participate, interact, and communicate (Handyside and Ringrose 2017; MacIsaac *et al.* 2018; Mascheroni, Vincent, and Jimenez 2015; Ringrose *et al.* 2013; Walsh 2017). It has also been reported that many young people use social media in a sexualised way, posting photos of their bodies that conform to normative sexualised stereotypes (Handyside and Ringrose 2017; Mascheroni, Vincent, and Jimenez 2015; Ringrose *et al.* 2013; Walsh 2017). While this content can be harmful by, for example, circulating images that have an affective influence on how others feel they should look and be (Ringrose *et al.* 2017), this self-focused behaviour also invites personal judgement, ridicule, and criticism (Handyside and Ringrose 2017; Mascheroni, Vincent, and Jimenez 2015). Furthermore, the images young people share of themselves and their bodies while, perhaps posted transiently, can take on an unanticipated 'life' (Handyside and Ringrose 2017). Similar to boyd's (2014) concept of visibility, Ringrose *et al.* (2013) reported that 'teen'-produced content can circulate widely and be used within peer networks as a form of digital currency. In turn, young people can become obsessed with the ways they look on social media, and it has been suggested that some are addicted to the feedback they obtain on whether their bodies conform to socially acceptable standards (Handyside and Ringrose 2017; Mascheroni, Vincent, and Jimenez 2015). In contrast to the more positive perspective of Ito *et al.* (2010) on the value of peer-based feedback, it is clear that research on gender and sexuality highlights some of the negative consequences of peer social media networks.

This brief overview has demonstrated that research from the fields of anthropology, psychology, and sociology has played an important part in advancing our understandings of the dynamic and interactive ways in which young people participate in social media. This work also emphasises the importance of understanding the issues and opportunities of digital media from young people's perspectives, and how participatory and ethnographic methods can generate new insights into learning, identity, media/digital literacy, ethics, and gender/sexuality. What is lacking from this perspective, however, is a specific focus on health and the ways in which young people's dynamic and interactive uses of social media shape their health-related knowledge and behaviours. Aside from Ito *et al.* (2010) there has also been a limited focus on learning, and there is a lack of understanding of the numerous factors that influence learning in a social media context. In the following section we consider the concept of pedagogy as a lens through which to interpret young people's health-related learning via social media. In addition to drawing upon existing understandings of pedagogy in health-related contexts, our research with young people and social media suggests that the concept of pedagogy could usefully be refined to fit the particular dynamism of social media. As a result, we propose some initial thoughts on the development of – what we have termed – a 'dynamic, content-led pedagogical framework'.

The case for reconsidering the concept of pedagogy in a social media context

Pedagogy provides a conceptual lens to frame the ways in which learning occurs in varied and diverse contexts (Armour 2014). 'Sport and Exercise Pedagogy' is one variation on the concept of pedagogy as translated into the field of physical education, physical activity, and health (Armour 2014; Armour and Chambers 2014) and technology-mediated learning in physical activity and health contexts (Casey *et al.* 2017, 2016). According to Armour and Chambers (2014, p. 858), sport and exercise pedagogy focusses on:

> (1) the needs of diverse learners of all ages in a wide range of physical activity/sport settings, including schools; (2) the abilities of professional teachers, coaches and instructors to meet those needs, and (3) the contexts in which relevant sport, exercise/health and physical education policy and knowledge are developed and delivered.

Sport and exercise pedagogy places young people's complex, diverse, and individual learning needs at its core (Armour 2014), and this focus aligns with the importance of understanding health-related social media from young people's perspectives. To date, however, the concept of sport and exercise pedagogy has been explored largely in formal contexts for learning, such as physical education or youth sport. It has also been argued that learning occurs at the moment where teaching/coaching practices, the curriculum, content/knowledge, and contexts align with and meet learners' needs (Armour 2014; Armour and Chambers 2014). Yet, in a social media context there is no defined teacher or curriculum and the contexts for learning are varied and shaped by multiple users and functionalities (Andersson and Olson 2014). As highlighted earlier in this chapter, social media is an informal context for learning and socialisation, where knowledge and behaviours can be influenced by diverse interactive functions (Walsh 2017), as well as by diverse people, who are either known (Ito *et al.* 2010) or unknown to individuals (James 2014). The concept of sport and exercise pedagogy is therefore limiting in framing learning within the dynamic and interactive context of social media.

Public pedagogies initially appeared to provide a neat umbrella concept to capture the informal learning context that characterises social media. Often grounded in the works of Giroux (2004), the concept of public pedagogies acknowledges learning as an experience that is influenced by popular culture (Burdick and Sandlin 2013). Giroux (2004) defined pedagogy as a political and moral practice, that represents the relationship between power, knowledge, and ideology (political) and how an individual invests in public life (moral). In turn, Giroux (2004) defined public pedagogy as the regulatory and emancipatory relationship between culture, power, and politics that occurs in a democratically configured social space. Giroux (2002) applied this concept of public pedagogy to explain how different forms of technology and media influence individuals' knowledge and behaviours, and this framework has been adopted widely in cultural and media studies (see Burdick and Sandlin 2013). For example, through particular representations in text, images, sounds, gestures, and dialogue, Giroux (2002, p. 539) argued that films operate pedagogically (i.e. politically and morally) through the 'common sense assumptions that inform them, the affective investments they mobilise, as well as the absence and exclusions that limit the range of meanings and information available'.

Similar to our challenges with applying the definition of sport and exercise pedagogy to social media data, connecting Giroux's conceptualisation of public pedagogies to contemporary digital media is problematic. For us, as for others, it was challenging to apply Giroux's concept that was grounded in a passive media context to an interactive and dynamic social media context (Andersson and Olson 2014; Andersson and Öhman 2017; Reid 2010). In particular, an analytical framing of pedagogy that operates through traditional conceptualisations of power seemed to neglect the role of young people in shaping content and educational experiences (Andersson and Olson 2014) and that is evident in, for example, boyd (2014) and Ito *et al.*'s (2010) concept of networked publics.

Returning to some of the anthropological framings of young people's experiences with social media (i.e. boyd 2014; Ito *et al.* 2010), the recent digital anthropological work of Miller and colleagues (Miller *et al.* 2016) was helpful to us in framing how pedagogy functions in a social media context (Goodyear *et al.* 2018a). Miller *et al.*'s (2016) focus in social media research has been based on content. Content is significant to Miller *et al.* (2016) because it migrates through social media platforms and is an enduring entity in the dynamism of online/digital media. Content, however, is not passive. Miller *et al.* (2016) suggest that content can be conceptualised as something users do, whereby content is actively constructed through different cultural genres (i.e. styles of use).

In addition to digital anthropology, Lomborg's (2011, 2017) research derived from communication theories was also helpful in understanding pedagogy in a dynamic social media context. Lomborg (2017) applied the concept of cultural genres to social media research to interpret the development of knowledge through communication. Lomborg (2017) – as well as Miller *et al.* (2016) – ground the concept of genres within the work of Goffman (1959), who argued that communication and sociality take place within cultural genres. In turn, Lomborg (2017) argued that genres provide analytical tools on the level of communicative practice. Genres are 'constituted by the interplay between interactive functionalities configured at the software level, and the invocation and appropriation of various software functionalities to achieve certain purposes, in and through users' actual communicative practices' (Lomborg 2017, n.p.).

By drawing on digital anthropology and communication theories, it was clear to us that an analytical framing of pedagogy in a social media context should be led by a focus on content. Content places the focus of analysis firmly on the active user and their interactions with content (Miller *et al.* 2016) and this focus aligned well with the research design that we adopted and that aimed to explain the data related to young people's perspectives (Goodyear *et al.* 2018a).

The data that we generated from young people about their engagement with health-related social media enabled us to pilot and develop the adapted conceptualisation of pedagogy (Goodyear *et al.* 2018a). The findings from this initial pilot work demonstrate that a content-led pedagogical framework can account for the very complex, dynamic, and interactive ways in which young people use social media, and can offer a framework to explain how young people's varying uses of social media influence their knowledge and behaviours (Goodyear *et al.* 2018a). Our content-led pedagogical framework, therefore, places content at its core (Figure 1.1) and can be understood as:

> The interplay between the user and the interactive functionalities of digital media: (i) leading to the construction of content, and (ii) shaping how content influences knowledge and understandings (Figure 1).
>
> (Goodyear *et al.* 2018a, p. 13)

The content-led pedagogical framework was used to analyse the data from the underpinning research, and construct five themes that are reported in the form of case study narratives in Chapters 2–6. This framework is still, however, in the very early stages of development. Although we are beginning to demonstrate that the framework can be used to explain digital engagement in different contexts – such as those related to health-related apps and online professional development courses – further development, application, and critical review is required. There is a need to ensure that a content-led pedagogical framework is robust, practical to use, and can meet the needs and demands of a range of researchers from different disciplines.

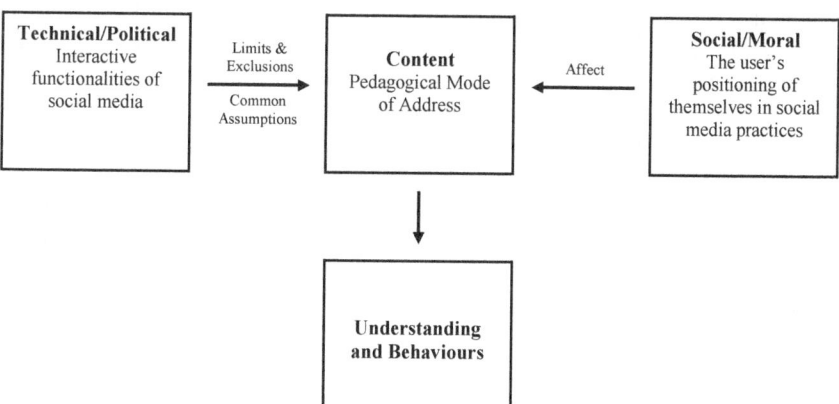

Figure 1.1 The operation of pedagogy in a social media context.

Source: Goodyear *et al.* 2018a, p. 13.

The structure and organisation of this book

The central method for illustrating and interpreting the ways in which young people's understandings of health and wellbeing both construct and are constructed by social media is *case study*. As has been demonstrated in previous books by the editors (see Armour 2014, 2003; Armour and Jones 1998; Casey *et al.* 2016; Jones *et al.* 2003), case studies offer a powerful mechanism to: (i) portray the lives, practices, and experiences of individuals, and (ii) to connect theory to practice (see also Thomas 2011) in ways that add new insights. The 'Pedagogical Cases' model created by Armour (2014) sought to crystallise the potential of case studies as a bridge between persisting research/theory-practice gaps. Armour (2014) drew on the seminal work of Stenhouse (1980) who advocated for case studies to support practitioner learning in education. Stenhouse was keen to *accumulate* case studies that could bridge theory and practice by developing a shared language about practice. Yet, although case studies do feature in most branches of educational research, there has been little attempt to accumulate them in the ways in which Stenhouse envisaged. The aspirations to bridge research/theory practice effectively are also largely unmet, with Ball (2012) pressing for the development of new communication channels, translational mechanisms, and resources. The development of pedagogical cases was an attempt to develop such a mechanism, and to ensure that single discipline research could better support the complex needs of interdisciplinary practice.

In previous books that have used the pedagogical cases model, multidisciplinary teams of academics have analysed fictional narratives of individual young people (Armour 2014) and co-constructed teacher narratives (Casey *et al.* 2016). In this book, the pedagogical case study model has been refined further and the core narratives are constructed from rich empirical data on young people (see detail below). The data are represented in composite narratives of young people that illustrate the key findings of the research, and contained within each narrative are responses by key stakeholders. The theoretical analyses are presented in separate chapters, similar to the approach used in the ground-breaking work by Connell (1986). Taken together, the narratives in each of the pedagogical case models offer a useful starting point for developing a bank of cases around which stakeholder learning can be organised.

In this book, six evidence-based composite narrative case studies have been constructed from the editors' funded research projects[2] undertaken with over 1,346 young people from the UK (as discussed in earlier sections of this chapter). What makes these case studies different from the previous pedagogical case books (see Armour 2014; Casey *et al.* 2016) is that each case study engages the voices of both young people and key stakeholders (e.g. schools, teachers, physical activity and health leaders in community settings, and policy and industry professionals). While case studies focused solely on young people (Armour 2014) and/or teachers and coaches (see Armour 2003; Armour and Jones 1998; Casey *et al.* 2016; Jones *et al.* 2003) provide rich narratives, they are limited in providing a 'complete picture' of physical activity and health education because the field crosses multiple settings. Social media is adding further complexity by increasing the diverse and easily accessible range of sources from which young people can learn about physical activity and health. It is interesting to note, for example, the absence of reference to physical education as a source of health education in the data from these young people (see Chapters 2–7).

In addition to composite case studies, this book follows the pedagogical cases model by offering insights into young people's uses of social media from diverse theoretical perspectives. As was noted earlier, theoretical analyses of young people and their engagement with social media have been undertaken predominantly in fields of anthropology, psychology, and sociology. Few connections between these theories have been made to date, and there have been very few theoretical insights into young people's uses of social media in the area of health and wellbeing. Given that social media has become an inherent part of young people's lives (boyd 2014; Turkle 2011), it is clear that this gap must be addressed, and this book represents an attempt to do just that. In Chapter 16, we summarise the contents of the book for multiple stakeholders and reflect on the effectiveness of the pedagogical case model in bridging the research-theory-practice divides, and the challenges of knowledge translation.

Chapter contents

In Chapters 2–7, composite narrative case studies of young people's engagement with health-related social media are presented. These chapters outline the different types of health-related content that young people access, create, and share on social media and that can influence their health-related knowledge and behaviours. The different types of content include:

- Automatically Sourced Content, that refers to the health-related information that social media sites pre-select and promote to young people (Kelly, Chapter 2).
- Suggested or Recommended Content, that refers to the process whereby young people's 'searches' for specific health-related information result in social media sites promoting vast amounts of partially related material to their accounts (Yaz, Chapter 3).
- Peer Content, that refers to the health-related content young people create, such as selfies (Leah, Chapter 4).
- Likes, that operate as a form of content through the process of affirmation (James, Chapter 5).
- Reputable Content, that refers to the power of specific social media accounts to frame the types of health-related information young people access and attend to (Jess, Chapter 6).

Chapter 7 presents a narrative case study of young people's recommendations and actions for adults. The chapter details how young people feel that different adults should support them to navigate health-related social media.

Chapters 8–15 provide a disciplinary analysis of the case study chapters from eight different disciplinary perspectives. Each of these chapters has a common format that includes: (i) a synthesis of existing research in the disciplinary area; (ii) case study analysis; and (iii) implications for supporting young people's engagement with health-related social media. These chapters focus on:

- *A salutogenic perspective:* outlining an alternative perspective on health that presents challenges to current policy, research and practice that is underpinned and often dominated by pathogenic perspectives. A salutogenic approach focuses on identifying new and diverse resources that young people draw on to support their health development. It is argued that social media can be a very powerful educative health resource (Quennerstedt, Chapter 8).
- *School physical education:* outlining how physical educators can contribute to young people's critical health literacy, develop pedagogies of affect, and deploy social media forms and content in critical and positive ways to support young people's health-related learning. This is an important contribution given the finding in the research that very few young people identified physical education as a source of health education (Kirk, Chapter 9).
- *Disordered eating:* outlines a continuum of problematic eating behaviours that ranges from unhealthy diets through to clinically diagnosed eating disorders, all of which can be influenced by content on social media. Valuable insights are provided into the important role of multi-component interventions to support young people's engagement with social media, including training for parents, teachers, school administrators, and local public health professionals, and where interventions are designed in collaboration with young people (Papathomas, White, and Plateau, Chapter 10).
- *Space, place and identity:* outlining the dualism between structure and agency in terms of how health is understood, portrayed, and performed in relation to social media. This is an important perspective that emphasises ways in which people's experiences of health-related social media are unique and varied based on differences in social landscapes (Sandford and Quarmby, Chapter 11).
- *Public pedagogies:* outlining how young people learn about their bodies, identities, and health through social media, and offering guidance as a counterbalance to the prevailing risk narrative. Recommendations are made on how to avoid technological determinism – that assumes social media is inherently oppressive or empowering – by focusing on embodied, affective learning in educational programmes (Rich, Chapter 12).
- *Health literacy:* outlining past and present public health agendas focused on developing patterns of health behaviours that transfer into adult life. This policy-informed perspective is vital to our understanding of young people and social media, and provides evidence of local and national interventions that can improve health literacy in response to social media content (Dudley, Van Bergen, McMaugh, and Mackenzie, Chapter 13).

- *Internet memes:* outlines how content is created, shared, and mobilised through the internet, and the problematic consequences of algorithms in determining what young people see, act upon, and use from social media. These cultural-technological insights are central to our understandings of how health-related knowledge and behaviours are formed by social media engagement (Casey, Chapter 14).
- *Digital democracy:* outlining the importance of student voice in pedagogical innovation. This chapter offers critical insights into how risk-based narratives can be navigated in health and physical education contexts. Youth participatory action research is presented as an alternative way of working with young people to help young people and adults engage with and learn about technology integration (Enright and Gard, Chapter 15).

Chapters 16–17 outline the new directions for research, policy, and practice that are based on the evidence that has been generated and presented from young people, key stakeholders, and diverse academic disciplines. In Chapter 16 we – Goodyear and Armour – evaluate whether the evidence, structure, and formatting of this book have been successful in providing policy makers, researchers, and health and education and practitioners/professionals with information that will help them to understand and better support young people's engagement with health-related social media. We do this by summarising the key findings for different stakeholder groups, and reflecting upon the value of the pedagogical cases framework and the challenges of engaging in successful knowledge translation and exchange. We also identify the further questions that the findings of this research raise. In Chapter 17 an independent analysis of the evidence and the book is provided by Cale. This final chapter outlines gaps in the existing evidence-base, limitations, and strengths of the book, and provides direction on the practices and/or interventions that will be effective in supporting, developing, and enhancing young people's health-related knowledge and behaviours.

Notes

1 The Wellcome Trust are a global charitable foundation, and are a UK-based research funding body. For further details, please see: https://wellcome.ac.uk/about-us
2 Details on the underpinning research funded by the Wellcome Trust can be accessed here: https://wellcome.ac.uk/what-we-do/directories/seed-awards-humanities-social-science-people-funded

References

Andersson, E. and Öhman, J., 2017. Young people's conversations about environmental and sustainability issues in social media. *Environmental Education Research*, 23, 465–485.

Andersson, E. and Olson, M., 2014. Political participation as public pedagogy – the educational situation in young people's political conversations in social media. *Journal of Social Science Education*, 13, 115–126.

Armour, K.M., 2014. *Pedagogical Cases in Physical Education and Youth Sport*. London: Routledge.

Armour, K.M. and Chambers, F.C., 2014. 'Sport and exercise pedagogy'. The case for a new integrative sub-discipline in the field of sport and exercise sciences/kinesiology/human movement sciences. *Sport, Education and Society*, 19, 855–868.

Armour, K.M. and Jones, R.L., 1998. *Physical Education Teachers' Lives and Careers: PE, Sport and Educational Status*. London: Routledge.

Ball, A.F., 2012. 2012 Presidential Address. To know is not enough: Knowledge, power and the zone of generativity. *Educational Researcher*, 41, 8, 283–293.

boyd, d., 2014. *It's Complicated: The Social Lives of Networked Teens*. London: Yale University Press.

boyd, d., 2007. Why youth (heart) social network sites: the role of networked publics in teenage social life. *In:* D. Buckingham, ed., *MacArthur Foundation Series on Digital Learning – Youth, Identity, and Digital Media*. Cambridge, MA: MIT Press, 119–142.

Buckingham, D., 2016. Is there a digital generation? *In:* D. Buckingham and R. Willett, eds. *Digital Generations: Children, Young People and the New Media*. London: Routledge, 1–18.

Burdick, J. and Sandlin, J.A., 2013. Learning, becoming, and the unknowable: Conceptualizations, mechanisms and processes in public pedagogy literature. *Curriculum Inquiry*, 43, 142–177.

Casey, A., Goodyear, V.A., and Armour, K.M., 2017. Rethinking the relationship between pedagogy, technology and learning in health and physical education. *Sport, Education and Society*, iFirst, 22(2), 288–304.

Casey, A., Goodyear, V.A., and Armour, K.M., 2016. *Digital Technologies and Learning in Physical Education: Pedagogical Cases*. London: Routledge.

Connell, R.W., 1986. *Teachers' Work*. London: George, Allen & Unwin.

Frith, E., 2017. Social media and children's mental health: A review of the evidence. Available from: from: https://epi.org.uk/wp-content/uploads/2017/06/Social-Media_Mental-Health_EPI-Report.pdf

Gaplin, A. and Taylor, G., 2017. Changing behaviour: Children, adolescents and screen use. Accessed from: www.bps.org.uk/sites/beta.bps.org.uk/files/Policy%20-%20Files/Changing%20behaviour%20-%20children%2C%20adolescents%2C%20and%20screen%20use.pdf

Gardner, H. and Davis, K., 2014. *The App Generation*. New Haven, CT: Yale University Press.

Giroux, H.A., 2004. Public pedagogy and the politics of neo-liberalism: Making the political more pedagogical. *Policy Futures in Education*, 2, 494–503.

Giroux, H.A., 2002. From 'Manchild' to 'Baby Boy': Race and the politics of self-help. *JAC*, 22, 527–560.

Goffman, E. 1959. *The Presentation of the Self in Everyday Life*. Garden City, NY: Anchor Books.

Goodyear, V.A., 2017. Social media, apps, and wearable technologies: Navigating ethical dilemmas and procedures. *Qualitative Research in Sport, Exercise and Health*, 9(3), 285–302.

Goodyear, V.A., Armour, K.M., and Wood, H., 2018a. Young people and their engagement with health-related social media: New perspectives. *Sport, Education and Society*, iFirst, doi:10.1080/13573322.2017.1423464.

Goodyear, V.A., Armour, K.M., and Wood, H., 2018b. *The Impact of Social Media on Young People's Health and Wellbeing: Evidence, Guidelines and Actions*. Birmingham, UK: University of Birmingham.

Graham, I.D., Logan, J., Harrison, M.B., Straus, S.E., Tetroe, J., Caswell, W., and Robinson, N., 2006. Lost in knowledge translation: Time for a map? *Journal of Continuing Education in the Health Professions*, 26, 13–24.

Handyside, S. and Ringrose, J., 2017. Snapchat memory and youth digital sexual cultures: Mediated temporality, duration and affect. *Journal of Gender Studies*, 26(3), 347–360.

Haussmann, J.D., Touloumtzis, C., White, M.T., Colbert, M.D., and Golding, H.C., 2017. Adolescent and young adult use of social media for health and its implications. *Journal of Adolescent Health*, 60(6), 714–719.

Highfield, T. and Leaver, T., 2017. Instagrammatics and digital methods: Studying visual social media, from selfies and GIFs to memes and emoji. *Communication Research and Practice*, 2 (1), 47–62.

Holmberg, C., Chaplin, E.J., Hillman, T., and Berg, C., 2016. Adolescents' presentations of food in social media: An explorative study. *Appetite*, 99, 121–129.

Hopkins, P.E., 2010. *Young People, Place and Identity*. Abingdon, Oxon: Routledge.

Inchley, J., Currie, D., Jewell, J., Breda, J., and Barnekow, V., eds., 2017. Adolescent obesity and related behaviours: Trends and inequalities in the WHO European Region, 2002–2014. *Observations from the Health Behaviour in School-aged Children (HBSC) WHO collaborative cross-national study*. Copenhagen, WHO Regional Office for Europe.

Ito, M., Baumer, S., Bittanti, M., boyd, d., Cody, R., *et al.*, 2010. *Hanging Out, Messing Around, and Geeking Out: Kids Living and Learning with New Media*. Cambridge, MA: MIT Press.

James, C., 2014. *Disconnected: Youth, New Media and the Ethics Gap*. London: MIT Press.

James, C., Davis, K., Flores, A., Francis, J.M., Pettingill, L., *et al.*, 2014. *Young People, Ethics, and the New Digital Media*. London: MIT Press.

Jones, R.L., Armour, K.M., and Potrac, P., 2003. *Sports Coaching Cultures: From Practice to Theory*. London: Routledge.

Jong, S.T. and Drummond, M.J.N., 2016. Hurry up and 'like' me: Immediate feedback on social networking sites and the impact on adolescent girls. *Asia-Pacific Journal of Health, Sport and Physical* Education, 7(3), 251–267.

Leahy, D., Burrows, L., McCuaig, L., Wright, J., and Penney, D., 2016. *School Health Education in Changing Times*. London: Routledge.

Livingstone, S., 2017. Children's and Young People's Lives Online. *In:* D. Brown, ed., *Online Risk to Children: Impact, Protection and Prevention*. London: Wiley Blackwell, 23–36.

Livingstone, S., Mascheroni, G., Ólafasson, K., and Haddon, L., 2014. *Children's Online Risks and Opportunities: Comparative Findings from EU Kids Online and Net Children Go Mobile*. London: London School of Economics and Political Science.

Livingstone, S., Mascheroni, G., and Staksrud, R., 2017. European research on children's internet use: Assessing the past and anticipating the future. *New Media & Society*, 20(3), 1103–1122.

Livingstone, S. and Third, A., 2017. Children and young people's rights in the digital age: An emerging agenda. *New Media & Society*, 19(5), 657–670.

Lomborg, S., 2017. *Social Media, Social Genres*. London: Routledge.

Lomborg, S., 2011. Social media as communicative genres. *Journal of Media and Communication Research*, 51, 55–71.

MacIsaac, S., Kelly, J., and Gray, S., 2018. 'She has like 4000 followers!': The celebrification of self within school social networks. *Journal of Youth Studies*,21(6), 816–835.

Mascheroni, G., Jorge, A., and Farrugia, L., 2014. Media representations and children's discourses on online risks: Findings from qualitative research in nine European countries. *Cyberpsychology: Journal of Psychosocial Research in Cyberspace*, 8(2), article 2.

Mascheroni, G., Vincent, J., and Jimenez, E., 2015. 'Girls are addicted to likes so they post semi-naked selfies': Peer mediation, normativity and the construction of identity online. Cyberspychology: *Journal of Psychosocial Research on Cyberspace*, 9(1), article 5.

Miller, D., Costa, E., Haynes, N., McDonald, T., Nicolescu, R., *et al.*, 2016. *How the World Changed Social Media.* London: UCL Press.

Oliver, K.M. and Kirk, D., 2016. Towards an activist approach to research and advocacy for girls and physical education. *Physical Education and Sport Pedagogy*, 21, 313–327.

Patton, G.C., Sawyer, S.M., Santelli, J.S., Ross, D.A., Afifi, R. *et al.*, 2016. Our future: A Lancet commission on adolescent health and wellbeing. *Lancet*, 387, 2423–2478.

Reid, A., 2010. Social media, public pedagogy and the end of private learning. *In:* J.A. Sandlin, B.D. Shultz, and J. Burdick, eds., *Handbook of Public Pedagogy*. London: Routledge, 194–200.

Ringrose, J., Harvey, L., Gill, R., and Livingstone, S., 2013. Teen girls, sexual double standards and 'sexting': Gendered value in digital image exchange. *Feminist Theory*, 14, 305–323.

Royal Society of Public Health., 2017. #*Status on Mind: Social Media and Young People's Mental Health and Wellbeing*. London: Royal Society for Public Health.

Shaw, J.M. Mitchell, C.A., Welch, A.J., and Williamson, M.J., 2015. Social media used as a health intervention in adolescent health: A systematic review of the literature. *Digital Health*, 1, 1–10.

Stenhouse, L., 1980. Presidential Address: The study of samples and the study of cases. *British Educational Research Journal*, 6, 1, 1–6.

Sparkes, A. and Smith, B., 2014. Ethical issues in qualitative research. *In:* A. Sparkes and B. Smith, eds., *Qualitative Research Methods in Sport, Exercise and Health: From Process to Product*. London: Routledge, 206–237.

Swist, T., Collin, P., McCormack, J., and Third, A., 2015. *Social Media and the Well-being of Children and Young People: A Literature Review*. Perth, WA: Prepared for the Commissioner for Children and Young People, Western Australia.

Third, A., Bellerose, D., Oliveira, J.D.D., Lala, G., and Theakstone, G., 2017. *Young and Online: Children's Perspectives on Life in the Digital Age*. Sydney: Western Sydney University.

Third, A., Bellerose, D., Dawkins, U., Keltie, E., and Pihl, K., 2014. *Children's Rights in the Digital Age: A Download from Children Around the World*. Melbourne: Young and Well Cooperative Research Centre.

Thomas, G., 2011. *How To Do Your Case Study*. London, Sage.

Turkle S. 2017. *Alone Together: Why We Expect More from Technology and Less from Each Other*. 3rd edn. New York: Basic Books.

Walsh, J., 2017. *Adolescents and Their Social Media Narratives*. London: Routledge.

Wartella, E., Rideout., V., Montague, H., Beaudoin-Ryan, L., and Lauricella, A., 2016. Teens, health, and technology: A national survey. *Media and Communications*, 4(3), 12–23.

Part I

Case studies of young people's engagement with health-related social media

2 Kelly

Automatically sourced social media content

Victoria A. Goodyear, Hannah Wood,
and Kathleen M. Armour

Chapter overview

This chapter introduces, illustrates, and analyses the finding that young people are open and vulnerable to rampant commercialism on social media. Data suggest that young people do not necessarily look or search for health-related information on social media, yet they see a significant number of health-related posts because of the algorithms embedded within social media sites and the unethical actions of commercial parties. This chapter argues that young people should be supported to develop deeper understandings of the algorithms embedded within social media and how these control and manipulate what young people can see, access, and use.

A digitally animated case study video of the evidence presented in this chapter can be accessed from: http://epapers.bham.ac.uk/3055/

Chapter structure and underpinning evidence

This chapter is organised into three main sections. In Section One, a narrative of a young person – Kelly – is presented to tell the story from the perspective of young people about the pervasive acts of commercialism found on social media. The narrative was constructed from an extensive data set (as detailed in Chapter 1) and it illustrates the voices and experiences of over 1,300 young people in the UK. Direct quotes from the data are shown in quotation marks. In Section Two – the stakeholder response – an interpretation of the narrative and recommended actions for research, policy, and practice are provided. The profile of the stakeholder group was international, multi-sector, and multi-disciplinary and included teachers, international academics (UK, Ireland, Sweden, Netherlands, Spain, Australia, China), and trusts/organisations in the UK (such as NHS, Youth Sport Trust) that have a focus on youth health and wellbeing. The stakeholder group watched a digital animated video of the case study narrative[1] and collaborated to produce the response during a one-day workshop (as detailed in Chapter 1). In Section Three, the key messages that emerge from the narrative and the stakeholder response are summarised.

Section One: young person's narrative – Kelly

A world without social media: 'are you mad?!'. Kelly has all the social media sites. She has Snapchat, Instagram, WhatsApp, YouTube, Facebook, Twitter, Tumblr … the list goes on. There isn't a social media site that she 'hasn't got an account on'. Kelly 'doesn't use them all' though, 'she just has the accounts'. She keeps them all so she can 'contact friends' and be contacted at any time. Social media is a good way to 'talk to people quickly'; 'especially about homework', and you 'can have great group chats'. *Kelly uses social media to communicate and so she can always be* **connected to her friends**.

Kelly mainly uses 'Snapchat and Instagram'. She said that 'everyone else had them' so she 'just followed everyone else'. Snapchat is the most popular. For Kelly, it's got to the stage now where if you 'haven't got Snapchat, it means you're a dead person'. Besides, 'no one ever texts nowadays'. Why text when you can 'just take a picture' and post it to Instagram or Snapchat a video? It's just easier, it's 'quick'. 'People our age mostly post images and videos and we only really look at images and videos'. *Kelly's use of social media is influenced by what* **everyone else does**, *and communication occurs through* **images and videos**.

When you can't be on Snapchat or Instagram you have to tell 'everyone else' why, otherwise they'll think you're ignoring them or that you're in a mood, and 'everyone else' will find out about it. So 'if you haven't got any Wi-Fi' or 'you haven't got data', you put 'no-reply'. 'If you're in a mood you put, not in the mood, no replies … NITM'. *Kelly has to post to social media to* **explain why she will be disconnected** *from her friends*.

Kelly's engagement with social media for health

Kelly doesn't associate social media with health; after all, she uses it primarily to stay *connected with her friends*. She doesn't post *images* or *videos* about her diet, her sleep, how she exercises, or any images of her body. Her friends don't either. This is 'personal' information and she just 'doesn't see the point'. Kelly wouldn't look for anything related to health on social media either. She hears enough about it at school, from her 'teachers' and in 'PE'. *Kelly would* **not post or look for** *anything related to health on social media*.

Kelly does, however, see *images and videos* on diet, sleep, exercises, and body image. 'Sponsored *videos* and pictures come up', sometimes just 'randomly'. The adverts are mainly from commercial brands, like 'Nike and Adidas'. There are also sponsored adverts on 'diets', 'vitamins', or these new types of 'water diets'. Kelly doesn't choose to see these health-related posts but they're 'everywhere'. The posts related to health are all over social media. Kelly *sees* **images and videos related to health**, even though she doesn't look for them.

Aside from the *sponsored adverts*, Kelly mainly *sees images and videos* related to health through the Search and Explore function on Instagram. She says 'on Instagram there's like this search page [Explore], so when you scroll down it's like just random things from anyone'. Yet 'loads of health' posts keep 'popping up', particularly the ones related to diets. Kelly *sees* these posts because of the algorithms embedded within Instagram. This is seen through the Explore button. The Explore button tailors what you see on Instagram based on the images the people you follow post, and/or the images the people you follow like.[2] In addition, Instagram says they also 'include posts from a mixture of hand-picked and automatically sourced accounts based on the topics we think you'll enjoy'. This means that the friends Kelly is connected to (i.e. those she follows) are either liking images or following other people outside of her peer network who post *images* about health. Instagram is also selecting the topics of posts that Kelly sees. *Kelly sees images and videos related to health because of the friends she is connected to and the automatically sourced accounts.*

Kelly says that she swipes past or just 'scrolls through' the *images and videos related to health*. Most of the time she doesn't think that their content is 'important for her age group' because 'people her age shouldn't be dieting'. Besides, the images send the wrong message and make it look as if there are 'shortcuts' to a healthy life. For example, although an advert says you can lose weight in '2 days', for others 'it might take 2 weeks'. Kelly **ignores** most of the health posts she sees, as they are **not appropriate for people her age**.

Kelly's friends to whom she is *connected* must be looking at images and videos related to diet drinks. 'Healthy' teas, coffees, and smoothies just 'come up'. Kelly 'doesn't choose to look at it', but they are just there when she goes onto Explore because of the algorithms of Search and Explore. Kelly can now explain what the 'healthy' teas are. She says FitTea 'is some tea that makes you healthy'. Kelly isn't exactly sure why it's healthy, but she thinks it's to do with 'protein in the tea'. But there are 'loads of different types' of these 'healthy teas' and they must be 'really popular', otherwise she wouldn't see them all the time or know what they are. *Kelly has **learned of a diet drink from social media** because of the friends she is connected to and the automatically sourced accounts.*

'Loads of people' at Kelly's school are now 'drinking green tea' and other 'types of healthy teas'. Kelly says that they have started 'taking things that are bad for the body' which can lead to things like 'anorexia'. Despite Kelly knowing the risks, she has started to copy what *everyone else does*. Because *everyone else* looks at stuff on Explore, she has started to pay more attention to the posts, adverts, and sponsored things she sees. Where previously she would not even entertain the idea of looking at health-related posts, she now says, 'I might take a look at them', even though 'they're not something I am searching for'. *Kelly now **looks at images and videos** related to health on social media because of the friends she **is connected to** and because it is what **everyone else does**. To **stop seeing** these videos and images, Kelly would need to **disconnect from her friends** on social media – which is unthinkable.*

Narrative summary

Kelly uses social media to communicate and so she can always be **connected to her friends**. The ways in which Kelly uses social media to communicate are influenced by what **everyone else does**, and mainly by her peers. For Kelly, and other young people her age, communication on social media primarily occurs through **images and videos**. The desire to be connected continuously to her friends through social media is apparent, particularly because Kelly feels she must post to social media to **explain why she will be disconnected** from her friends; that is, when she won't be on social media. Kelly would **not post or look for** anything related to health on social media. However, Kelly **sees images and videos related to health**, even though she also doesn't look for them. Kelly sees images and videos related to health because of **the friends she is connected to on social media and automatically sourced accounts**. Kelly **ignores** most of the health posts she sees because she is aware that they are **not appropriate for people of her age**. Yet, Kelly has **learned about a diet drink from social media** because of the friends she is connected to and automatically sourced accounts. Kelly now **looks at** images and videos related to health on social media because of the friends she is **connected to** and because it is what **everyone else does**. To stop seeing these videos and images, Kelly would need to **disconnect from her friends** on social media – which is unthinkable.

Section Two: stakeholder response

Social media can have a positive impact on young people's health and wellbeing because it increases and strengthens the opportunities young people have to *sustain* and *develop* peer relations. At the same time, the desire to stay constantly connected to peers on social media – as seen in Kelly's narrative – leaves young people open and vulnerable to a range of pervasive acts of commercialism. This exposure can impact negatively on young people's health-related behaviours, including diet/nutritional intake and body image perception. To address these risk-related impacts, young people need to develop deeper understandings of the algorithms used in social media and how these control and manipulate what young people can see, access, and use. Young people also need to develop critical skills to navigate the potentially unethical actions of commercial parties.

Sustaining and developing peer relations

Social media can be a powerful platform to support young people to *sustain* and *develop new peer relations*. Given that peer relations are frequently associated with health and wellbeing, the case study narrative illustrates a potentially positive impact of social media use on young people's social and emotional wellbeing. In particular, through social media, Kelly is able to sustain her contact with peers through easy and quick interactions. For example, by viewing the videos and images that Kelly posts to social media, Kelly's peers are able to gain deeper understandings of her personal, social, and emotional wellbeing. As a result, Kelly's peers could have an enhanced capacity to offer/provide social and emotional support to meet Kelly's needs at any point in time.

Social media also has the capacity to support young people to *develop* new peer relations through the ease of access to an expansive peer network. For example, the Search and Explore function enabled Kelly to see images and videos posted by people whom she did not know personally, but who clearly shared similar interests. This broad, yet personalised network has the potential to benefit young people by providing them with increased opportunities to collaborate and learn from others.

Easy commercial targets

Young people are easy commercial targets on social media. It would appear that both young people and adults are somewhat naïve about the unethical actions of commercial parties. Young people are particularly vulnerable to the pervasive health-related marketing strategies and subliminal commercial messaging that appear on social media. In other words, young people and adults often fail to appreciate that the reason health-related material reaches them – even though they have not actively searched for it – is because commercial parties have 'invaded' their social media peer networks.

Kelly's experiences of using Instagram highlight that commercial parties are highly skilled in manipulating the content young people consume and reproduce. Companies such as FitTea ensure that their products reach young people through increased visibility, generated by invading young people's social media peer networks. In addition, commercial parties use meta-data to 'ping' certain products to young people and to place sponsored adverts onto their timelines. These actions could be regarded as unethical given that they ruthlessly target young people for commercial gain.

The constant invasion of young people's social media networks by commercial parties is a clear risk for young people's health and wellbeing. Kelly's experiences highlight how young people can be trapped in an endless cycle of consuming and producing inappropriate health-related products simply because they are present in a wide online peer network. The narrative indicates that these posts can lead to potentially harmful health-related products being accepted as 'healthy', and that young people are too trusting, with the potential outcome that some could act unwisely on the basis of largely unregulated information.

Considerations

*Unfettered access to social media is regarded by young people as a
'right' that is also essential for their wellbeing*

Engaging with social media and using digital technologies are a *way of living* for young people. Numerous sites, apps, and devices are used multiple times a day and are woven into the very fabric of contemporary youth culture. Young people primarily use social media to stay connected to their friends and this connectedness could be regarded as a positive influence on their social and emotional wellbeing. It is, perhaps, unsurprising that young people regard unfettered access to social media as a 'right'.

Young people and adults need to be better informed about the risk-related impacts of social media on young people's health and wellbeing

When young people use and engage with social media they encounter significant amounts of unsolicited and unregulated health-related material, and this can result in harm. To address these risks, both young people and adults need a deeper understanding of the ways in which commercial interests use social media to control and manipulate what young people see and access, and enhanced critical skills to help them to navigate this commercial invasion of their digital spaces. There are clear opportunities for schools/teachers and parents/guardians to support young people to be more critically aware of the information they see and access. The development of evidence-based constructivist and experiential learning tasks could be one way forward, but it has to be recognised that most adults are out of their depth in the digital spaces inhabited by youth; and young people are very aware of this. Adults themselves require new forms of support so that they are in a better position to support young people more effectively.

Section Three: key messages from the case

This case has identified that although young people do not necessarily look or search for health-related information on social media, they see a significant number of health-related posts because of the algorithms embedded within social media sites and the unethical actions of commercial parties. The case suggests that young people should be supported to develop deeper understandings of the algorithms used in social media and how these control and manipulate what young people can see, access and use. A summary of the key messages from the case can be found in Table 2.1.

Table 2.1 Key messages about automatically sourced content

Characteristics of Young People's Uses of Social Media for Health	Young people use social media to communicate and to stay connected to their peers. Many young people would not post or look for anything related to health on social media. Yet, young people see images and videos related to health because of the algorithms embedded within social media, such as automatically sourced accounts. While many young people ignore most of the health posts they see – as they understand that they are not appropriate for people their age – some young people begin to learn about the health-related products that are promoted to them through their peer networks, and by the algorithms. To stop seeing these videos and images, young people would need to disconnect from their friends on social media – which is unthinkable.
Stakeholder Response Focused on Young People's Uses of Social Media for Health	Social media can be a powerful platform to support young people to sustain and develop new peer relations. At the same time, young people are vulnerable to the pervasive health-related marketing strategies and subliminal commercial messaging that appear on social media. Posts made by commercial parties can influence young people to engage in harmful health-related behaviours, that can be inappropriate for their stage of development.
Considerations for Research, Policy, and/or Practice	Unfettered access to social media is regarded by young people as a 'right' and is also essential for their wellbeing. Young people and adults need to be better informed about the risk-related impacts of social media on young people's health and wellbeing.

Notes

1 The digital animated case study narrative video of Kelly can be accessed here: http://epapers.bham.ac.uk/3055/
2 Search & Explore: We're always working to update the types of photos and videos you see in Search & Explore to better tailor it to you. Posts are selected automatically based on things like the people you follow or the posts you like. You may also see video channels, which can include posts from a mixture of hand-picked and automatically sourced accounts based on topics we think you'll enjoy: https://help.instagram.com/487224561296752

3 Yaz

Suggested or recommended social media content

Victoria A. Goodyear, Hannah Wood,
and Kathleen M. Armour

Chapter overview

This chapter introduces, illustrates, and analyses the finding that health-related information that young people perceive to be relevant to their needs is highly accessible on social media. However, most of the health-related material available to young people could be regarded as inappropriate, as it is designed for and targeted at adult populations. This chapter argues that social media designers have a responsibility to protect young people from inappropriate health-related content that is easily accessible. Schools/teachers and parents/guardians also have a responsibility to empower young people to act critically, safely, and ethically in digital/online environments, while also developing their health literacy.

A digitally animated case study video of the evidence presented in this chapter can be accessed from: http://epapers.bham.ac.uk/3062/

Chapter structure and underpinning evidence

This chapter is organised into three main sections. In Section One, a narrative of a young person – Yaz – is presented to tell the story from young people's perspectives about the potential impact of easily accessible health information. The narrative was constructed from an extensive data set (as detailed in Chapter 1) and illustrates the voices and experiences of over 1,300 young people in the UK. Direct quotes from the data are shown in quotation marks. In Section Two – stakeholder response – an interpretation of the narrative and recommended actions for research, policy, and practice are provided. The profile of the stakeholder group was international, multi-sector, and multi-disciplinary and included teachers, international academics (UK, Ireland, Sweden, Netherlands, Spain, Australia, China), and trusts/organisations in the UK (such as NHS, Youth Sport Trust) that have a focus on youth health and wellbeing. The stakeholder group watched a digital animated video of the case study narrative[1] and collaborated to produce the response during a one-day workshop (as detailed in Chapter 1). In Section Three, the key messages that emerge from the narrative and the stakeholder response are summarised.

Section One: young person's narrative – Yaz

Yaz has always 'turned to the internet to search for things'. But he says social media is *so* much better. Like on YouTube, you don't have to search for the information you want because they have videos 'suggested for you'. These videos are based on similar videos to those you have watched previously and they just 'come up' on your home page. The videos play on an 'infinite loop' and you can find out 'loads' of different pieces of information about the same topic. Yaz says the videos are 'really helpful' because they are 'relatable' to you. Relevant information just finds you! *Social media provides Yaz with **access** to **information** that he perceives to be **helpful** because it is **relatable** to him and relevant to his needs.*

The videos Yaz watches on YouTube help him 'learn how to do stuff'. Compared to websites, social media doesn't give you 'information essays'. The videos are 'easy to understand' and 'straight to the point'. You can look in like 'two minutes'; sometimes in just '2 seconds'. Yaz says he doesn't have time to look through a lot of stuff because of all the 'homework' he gets – especially with 'exams' coming up, so the videos relate to his needs. *Information accessed from social media helps Yaz to **learn** because it is **easy to understand, straight to the point** and **relevant to his needs**.*

Yaz's engagement with social media for health

Yaz is interested in physical activity videos on YouTube. Yaz has found the physical activity campaigns on YouTube's 'suggested for you' page 'intriguing'. These campaigns are run by official health organisations and aim to get more people active. Campaigns like '#ThisGirlCan'[2] or the 'Dove Campaign'.[3] Yaz has watched the campaign videos over and over again on the 'infinite loop' of 'suggested' videos. He says these campaigns are 'quite inspiring' for girls. Some girls at his school have a new found 'motivation' for physical activity. The campaigns are effective because girls can *relate* to them. The girls say that you get to see 'real people' doing exercise and you can watch 'the actual reality of people doing exercise'. Yaz's friend, Amy, said that one of the campaigns showed her that 'it wasn't just her who looked like an absolute slob when she runs' and it made her 'want to exercise'. Even when the campaigns ended, Amy, who is not very active, was 'motivated to continue exercising'. But there are hardly any campaigns for boys; they are all targeted at girls. *Physical activity campaigns on social media **motivate** girls Yaz's age to be physically active because the girls can **relate to** the real people in the videos.*

Within the 'infinite loop' of 'suggested' and 'recommended' videos on YouTube, Yaz has been able to *learn* about the transformations that can happen to your body when you engage in physical activity. There are lots of 'transformation' videos of people. The exercises say things such as: you 'get the body you want', and they show 'before and after' transformations. He says that the videos show 'people taking pictures of their muscles and stuff' and they caption the videos with things 'like gains and that'. Even though the people uploading the transformation videos are in their 'early 20s' Yaz can *relate* to them. Like other boys his age, Yaz wants to be more 'muscley' and 'buff'. He says the videos 'kind of inspire him to be better' and they 'motivate' him 'to work on his body'. He sees the transformations videos and thinks: 'I want to do that. I want to build'. *Yaz relates to the people in the **body trans-** **formation videos** because he wants to be more muscular and he has been **inspired** to engage with the **muscle-gaining exercises** that are 'suggested' and 'recommended' to him.*

On the 'suggested for you' page there are lots of 'bodybuilding' and 'weight training' videos. You can't escape them. Yaz has been particularly interested in the 'no pain, no gain' videos. These videos clearly relate to 'loads' of people as they have more than 100 likes and that shows 'appeal'. If something has less than 100 likes 'it doesn't show appeal' and that 'other people aren't interested, so why should you be'. So Yaz thinks that 'loads of people' must be doing the exercises in the videos, even though they are about 'older' people. After all, they are also 'trending' on YouTube. So Yaz has started to believe in 'no pain, no gain'. The motto is 'straight to the point' and it's 'easy to understand'. When he exercises, Yaz says he keeps in the back of his mind the thought that 'if you don't push yourself enough, you won't get past the pain'. *Yaz perceives that the videos he sees on YouTube **relate to a wide audience**, so he has started to **act on the information** he sees on YouTube when he **exercises in the gym**.*

Yaz's friend Amy is concerned. She thinks that social media has pressured Yaz into being a 'fitness fanatic' and that the workouts 'strain him too much'. Amy is aware that copying 'adults just going to the gym' can give you 'weird muscles'. She says that your 'bodies aren't going to be developed enough'. It can 'stunt your growth'. Amy understands what Yaz is doing because she was motivated to engage in the social media physical activity campaigns. But the videos don't relate to Yaz, even though he thinks they do. They are for 'older people' and Amy thinks that Yaz has now gone too far. *The information on the videos could be **harmful** for Yaz's **physical development**. In doing the exercises that were 'suggested' and 'recommended', he was beginning to strain his body too much and he was becoming a **fitness fanatic**.*

Narrative summary

Social media provides Yaz with **access** to **information** that is **helpful** because he perceives it to be **relatable** to him. Information accessed from social media helps Yaz to **learn** because it is **easy to understand**, **straight to the point**, and **is relevant to his needs**. Yaz is aware of physical activity campaigns on social media that are targeted at girls. These physical activity campaigns **motivate** girls Yaz's age to be physically active because the girls can **relate to** the real people in the videos. Yaz, however, relates to the people in the **body transformation**

videos because these are more tailored to his needs. Yaz wants to be more muscular and he has been **inspired** to engage with the **muscle-gaining exercises** that are 'suggested and recommended to him' on YouTube. Yaz also perceives that the videos he sees on YouTube **relate to a wide audience**, so he has started to **act on the information** he sees on YouTube when he **exercises in the gym**. It was apparent that some of the information in the videos could be **harmful** for Yaz's **physical development**. In doing the exercises that were 'suggested' and 'recommended', he was beginning to strain his body too much and he was becoming a **fitness fanatic**.

Section Two: stakeholder response

Social media can result in young people developing narrow understandings of health. The algorithmic properties embedded within social media sites limit access to a wider and more diverse range of health-related information, and this constrains the development of a broad understanding of health. Young people are also particularly receptive and vulnerable to health-related material made available on social media, because young people perceive it to be relevant to their needs. As body awareness becomes a growing issue in adolescence, social media content related to health becomes increasingly interesting to young people. To help young people navigate the health-related spaces of social media, social media companies have a responsibility to protect young people from inappropriate content that is made easily accessible on social media. Schools/teachers and parents/guardians should also empower young people to act critically, safely, and ethically in digital/online environments, while also developing health literacy.

Algorithms

It is clear that the algorithms embedded within existing social media sites can contribute to promoting narrow understandings of health. A narrow understanding of health is often represented in the associations made between body shape and health; for example, slender is 'healthy' and fat is 'unhealthy'. The way that information is presented through the 'suggested for you' videos on YouTube shows how social media can intensify the acceptance of these narrow understandings of health. In the narrative, it was apparent that health was understood as being related to body shape, and this understanding was largely shaped by the information that was available, accessible, and 'suggested'. It was also clear that the 'suggested' content influenced physical activity behaviours. It can be argued that 'suggested' or 'recommended' content is influencing young people to develop a narrow understanding of health and also restricts their physical activity behaviours because the content is underpinned by a focus on body image.

The 'suggested' videos are based on similar topics to the videos an individual has viewed previously. In the narrative, Yaz was initially interested in different types of physical activity videos. Yaz viewed videos that focused on motivation and/or cardiorespiratory exercise (ThisGirlCampaign), and weight training and/or body building exercises. As Yaz became more interested in weight training and/or body building exercises, he began to view fewer videos focused on motivation and/or cardiorespiratory exercise. The algorithmic properties embedded within YouTube supported his growing interest in weight training and body building. As a result, Yaz no longer viewed different types of physical activity videos and he couldn't escape the weight training/body building videos. In this sense, Yaz's ability to be critical of the ideals of health promoted by the weight training or body building videos was constrained because YouTube failed to ensure that alternative physical activity videos were easily accessible to Yaz. In turn, Yaz became trapped in the idea that health equates to body shape, and was unable to critique the harmful physical activity behaviours he had adopted. Peer support from Amy, who recognised and understood how Yaz's physical activity behaviours were impacted by social media, appeared to be vital. It would have been interesting to learn if and how Amy confronted Yaz and what the outcomes of this peer support were.

Receptive = vulnerable

The narrative clearly shows that young people are receptive to health-related material available on social media. Adolescence is an age when young people become increasingly aware of their bodies. At the same time, it is widely apparent that social media use grows during the period of adolescence. In combination, an awareness of the body and increased social media use act as powerful incentives for young people to accept new suggestions and ideas from social media about their bodies and health. This level of receptivity to material from social media makes young people vulnerable. The similar ways in which Amy and Yaz accessed and acted on social media material highlights the fact that these young people were receptive and vulnerable at the same time.

Amy and Yaz were both receptive to videos about physical activity that were available on YouTube. Although they acted on different types of physical activity information (cardiorespiratory vs muscle gain), Amy and Yaz both accessed information that could result in harm. Specifically, they acted on information that was primarily targeted at adults,[4] and was neither age nor developmentally appropriate. Their willingness to use information targeted at adults to inform their physical activity behaviours illustrates how both Yaz and Amy were vulnerable.

As negative impacts on Yaz's physical development were identified, one reading of the narrative would be that Yaz was more vulnerable than Amy. The lack of critique employed by Amy on the adult-focused material she accessed and acted on, however, suggests that she was equally vulnerable. While Amy's health was positively impacted, through an increased level of motivation for physical activity, Amy acted on material that was developed for and targeted at adults. Amy only considered the inappropriateness of using such material when Yaz's behaviour became addictive and obsessive, and his body shape and size had changed dramatically. In this sense, inappropriate social media material was only critiqued and identified and disregarded as 'healthy' when offline behaviour and appearance displayed negative impacts.

The narrative exemplifies the importance of focusing on the discrete skills practiced by all young people on social media and how social media has the potential to intensify young people's vulnerability. In addition, the narrative shows that young people need to acquire a level of health literacy; that is, to be supported to develop an understanding of information that is relevant to their health-related needs.

Considerations

Technology companies and designers of social media sites have a responsibility to act ethically in order to limit the range of inappropriate health-related material that reaches young people

Minimum standards should be developed and applied to protect young people from inappropriate content that is 'suggested' and/or 'recommended' to them, and this would reduce the amount that reaches them through social media. Minimum standards would include a requirement for social media sites to apply account filters to regulate the ways in which information is advertised, marketed, and distributed to young people. In addition, all social media material about diet/ nutrition, exercise/physical activity, and body image material should include clear signposting that explains for whom the material is relevant/appropriate. As an example, a clear indication of the age-appropriateness of specific exercises could be provided. Ultimately, technology companies and designers of social media sites have a responsibility to deliver a service to young people that is safe, even if it is not in their immediate commercial interests.

Schools/teachers and parents/guardians have a responsibility to empower young people to act critically, safely, and ethically in digital/ online environments, while also developing their health literacy

Young people have a right to grow up as knowledgeable, practical, and empowered digital citizens who are able to understand digital social norms and manage risk for themselves. They need to be empowered to engage in critical, safe, and ethical behaviours. Young people should be supported to act prudently and carefully, and to become thoughtful users of social media. Equally, their health literacy should be developed in the context of their uses of social media. Young people needed to be supported to understand the types of health-related information that is relevant to their health-related needs. This is an important action/ responsibility for schools/teachers and parents/guardians.

Table 3.1 Key messages about suggested and recommended content

Characteristics of Young People's Uses of Social Media for Health	Health-related information is highly accessible to young people on social media. Young people can search for information, and they find health-related information from the algorithms that 'suggest' or 'recommend' content to their accounts. Young people engage with health-related information if they perceive it to be relevant to their needs. Some of the health-related information can be helpful and can motivate young people to engage with physical activity. Some of the content, however, can be harmful, particularly that related to body transformations and the type of content that is targeted at adult populations.
Stakeholder Response Focused on Young People's Uses of Social Media for Health	Algorithms embedded within social media sites can contribute to promoting narrow understandings of health for young people.
	A narrow understanding of health often equates health to body image. For example, slender is healthy, fat is unhealthy.
	Young people are highly receptive to health-related information on social media, due to their age and excessive use of social media platforms.
Considerations for Research, Policy, and/or Practice	Technology companies and designers of social media sites have a responsibility to act ethically in order to limit the range of inappropriate health-related material that reaches young people.
	Schools/teachers and parents/guardians have a responsibility to empower young people to act critically, safely, and ethically in digital/online environments, while also developing their health literacy.

Section Three: key messages from the case

This case has identified that health-related information that young people perceive to be relevant to their needs is highly accessible to them on social media. The case suggests that social media designers have a responsibility to protect young people from inappropriate health-related content that is 'suggested' or 'recommended' to young people on social media. Schools/teachers and parents/guardians also have a responsibility to empower young people to act critically, safely, and ethically in digital/online environments, while also developing their health literacy.

Notes

1 The digital animated case study narrative video of Yaz can be accessed here: http://epapers.bham.ac.uk/3062/
2 www.thisgirlcan.co.uk
3 www.dove.com/uk/stories/campaigns.html
4 Although the ThisGirlCan campaign is targeted at women age 14–40, the stakeholders did not consider the key promotion videos and images to include or reflect young people. The campaign was positioned as an adult only campaign.

4 Leah

Peer content

Victoria A. Goodyear, Hannah Wood,
and Kathleen M. Armour

Chapter overview

This chapter introduces, illustrates, and analyses the finding that peer content (such as selfies) has a powerful influence on young people's levels of body satisfaction. Some young people are critical of peer content. At the same time, other young people experience a level of peer pressure to modify their health-related behaviours to look a certain way. The chapter argues that social media is a powerful educational resource that can open up dialogue about the body. Resilience can be developed by supporting young people to engage with peer content and by encouraging peers to offer support and critical insights.

A digitally animated case study video of the evidence presented in this chapter can be accessed from: http://epapers.bham.ac.uk/3061/

Chapter structure and underpinning evidence

This chapter is organised into three main sections. In Section One a narrative of a young person – Leah – is presented to tell the story from young people's perspectives about the ways in which social media intensify the opportunities for peer comparison. The narrative was constructed from an extensive data set (as detailed in Chapter 1) and illustrates the voices and experiences of over 1,300 young people in the UK. Direct quotes from the data are shown in quotation marks. In Section Two – stakeholder response – an interpretation of the narrative and recommended actions for research, policy, and practice are provided. The profile of the stakeholder group was international, multi-sector, and multi-disciplinary and included teachers, international academics (UK, Ireland, Sweden, Netherlands, Spain, Australia, China), and trusts/organisations in the UK (such as NHS, Youth Sport Trust) that have a focus on youth health and wellbeing. The stakeholder group watched a digital animated video of the case study narrative[1] and collaborated to produce the response during a one-day workshop (as detailed in Chapter 1). In Section Three, the key messages that emerge from the narrative and the stakeholder response are summarised.

Section One: young person's narrative – Leah

Leah says she uses social media 'every second' of 'everyday'. On Instagram she *follows* 'meme accounts', 'football accounts' and, as she is a big Aston Villa fan – she *follows* all the 'Villa Players'. However, Leah says that the point of using Instagram is for 'mainly just your friends' and to follow your 'friends'. By using social media Leah can always see what her friends are doing. Most of the things that she likes on Instagram are 'friends' posts', and she is far more likely to re-gram (re-share) one of her friend's posts than a post made by a celebrity. *Leah follows accounts outside her peer network, but the main purpose of using social media is to **look at and share her friends' posts**.*

Leah's engagement with social media for health

Leah's friends post to Instagram all the time. They post about 'everything', literally 'everything'. They post things like 'I woke up today, this is my breakfast' or just 'if they are going out'. Because Leah's friends post to social media all the time, she always knows what they are doing. Some of the boys post pictures of themselves 'being in the gym' with '#gymlad' or '#gains'. Some of the girls post pictures in their 'bikinis'. If they have a 'good figure' then they want to 'show it off'. Leah doesn't post Instagram pictures of herself though. She 'feels very self-conscious about her body' and 'wonders how people will react'. She doesn't think that her figure is 'what people want to see' and fears others might 'mock it'. *Leah's friends that she follows post **images of themselves in the gym or of their bodies, to show off.** Yet, Leah **does not post images of her body** because she feels too **self-conscious** and wants to **avoid potential ridicule**.*

Leah thinks that the 'skinny girls' are the worst. The 'skinny girls' aren't girls that Leah is friends with, but she follows them on Instagram. The 'skinny girls' are a similar age, and she sometimes sees them at school. Leah says that the 'skinny girls' are the type of girls who post to social media to 'find out what people think of them'. These girls know that their figures are 'better than others' and they just do it for 'attention'. They often caption their images with 'chunky monkey' or 'my thighs are big, damn it'. They say, 'oh, I'm so fat, I'm so fat' and 'they're literally like super skinny'. Leah says that the 'skinny girls' are always 'saying bad stuff about their figures' and they are constantly 'sticking out their pelvis' in photos, 'pretending to be fat'. The thing is, 'they clearly know their figure isn't that bad, otherwise they wouldn't have posted the picture in the first place'. *Leah sees posts made by other girls her age of their bodies, and these are often 'skinny girls' with good figures. Leah thinks these 'skinny girls' post to social media for **attention** and to **find out what people think of them**.*

Leah is 'really pissed' with the 'skinny girls'. She says that they just think about themselves and they don't realise how 'posting one picture can make someone feel insecure about themselves'. Leah looks at the 'skinny girls'' posts and thinks that her own figure 'is 10 times worse'. It makes Leah feel that she is 'not adequate' or not 'good enough'. She says that what the skinny girls post puts 'pressure on you' to look a certain way. For some young people it can be really bad. They might feel 'so pressured and obsessed to be that way that they might get unhealthy', 'maybe anorexic'. *The skinny girls Leah follows **don't** think about the impact of their posts on others and how their posts could lead others to suffer **emotional and physical harm**.*

Leah sees 'loads' of posts on Instagram of celebrities who are 'skinny' or who have 'perfect' 'hour glass figures'. But because the 'skinny girls' are 'her age' and 'she knows them', it makes her feel worse. It makes you feel like 'oh, I want to look like that'. Leah knows it's a form of 'peer pressure' and the images are wrong, but she can't escape it. It's different from being face-to-face at school; its 'proper peer pressure'. It's a 'bigger problem than cyber bullying', she says. 'Cyber bullying is a lot more noticeable than peer pressure'. You can see cyber bullying, through the comments. But the images you see are a 'bigger' form of peer pressure. It can 'make you think that you should do something' in order to look a certain way. Leah feels as though *the images posted by the skinny girls are a powerful form of **peer pressure** and it **makes her feel that she should do something to look a certain way**.*

Leah Snapchatted her friend Chloe about the 'skinny girls'' posts and how they 'basically just want attention'. Chloe replied by telling Leah that her attacks on the skinny girls make Chloe 'feel really uncomfortable' because she is 'naturally really slim'. Chloe tells Leah that people are always saying to her 'oh, you're too skinny, you need to eat more'. It makes Chloe feel that people 'just don't like her body'. Chloe says that this isn't fair because 'it's not like skinny is the kind of body that she wants'. Chloe adds, your body shape 'is not something that you can really help'. Chloe sympathises with the skinny girls and she tells Leah to think how 'people read posts in different ways'. Chloe suggests that the 'skinny girls' might not be posting to social media for attention, as Leah thinks. *Leah's friend Chloe responds to the skinny girls posts in a different way. Chloe sympathises with the skinny girls and she encourages Leah to look at the 'skinny girls' post in a different way and to think differently about how people making posts to social media may feel.*

Narrative summary

Leah uses social media to **look at and share her friends' posts**. Leah's friends that she follows post **images of themselves in the gym or of their bodies, to show off**. Leah **does not post images** of her body because she feels **too self-conscious** and wants to **avoid potential ridicule**. Skinny girls, that often have good figures, tend to post images of their bodies the most. Leah thinks that these girls post images of their bodies for attention and to **find out what people think of them**. The images posted by the skinny girls are a powerful form of **peer pressure** and it **makes Leah feel that she should do something to look a certain way**. Leah thinks that the skinny girls **don't think about the impact of their posts on others**. Yet Leah's friend – Chloe – sympathises with the skinny girls, and highlights that the girls might not be posting for attention. Chloe encourages Leah to look at the 'skinny girls'' post in a different way and to think differently about how people making posts to social media may feel.

Section Two: stakeholder response

Young people's constant exposure to images of bodies shared by peers on social media encourages peer comparison and this can lead to heightened levels of body dissatisfaction. To address potentially negative impacts, young people need to be supported to develop their resilience to these forms of peer content. Resilience can be developed through supporting young people to be empathetic towards the material posted by peers and by celebrating diversity in different body shapes and sizes. In this sense, social media is a powerful educational resource and should be used to open up dialogue about health and the body. Peer-to-peer support is also vital for young people, and schools/teachers and parents/guardians should ensure that appropriate pathways for peer support are in place.

Peer comparison

Social comparison is a common and expected behaviour of young people of a similar age to Leah. Young people often seek out and use information from others as a way to learn about how they should be and act. In many respects, social comparison is an activity that should be encouraged and supported – rather than prevented – as it is key to young people's development. Social comparison is a fundamental activity from which young people learn and find their place in society.

The narrative highlights the negative consequences of social comparison as a result of the information young people access and attend to on social media. For Leah, comparing her body to others who were of the same age but of a different shape and size led to feelings that are associated with body dissatisfaction. *Peer-to-peer body comparison* on social media can therefore be interpreted as a risky behaviour. As Leah suggested, peer-to-peer body comparison had a much more powerful influence on her levels of body dissatisfaction than celebrities or other individuals who were not of a similar age. Comparing oneself to others who are of the same age, gender, similar context or school, is extremely powerful. As a result, peer-to-peer comparison on social media is likely to be unhelpful for some young people in their efforts to construct nuanced understandings about how to be healthy.

The new understandings this narrative generates go beyond the issues of social or peer-to-peer body comparison, despite this being the strongest message. We know a lot about the negative consequences of social and peer comparison from a relatively large international evidence-base. The new message is that social media intensifies the experience of peer-to-peer body comparison. Through large peer networks and as a result of being constantly connected to social media (as evident in Chapter 2), young people are exposed to more images, photos, and videos of their peers' bodies than has been previously possible in face-to-face environments. This increased exposure to peer content increases the levels of peer-to-peer comparison and, for some young people, this is likely to be a harmful consequence of engaging with social media.

Resilience

Young people are not going to abandon their phones or stop using social media; these activities are woven into the very fabric of contemporary youth culture. At the same time, it is impractical for adults to continuously monitor social media use in an effort to address risky behaviours. Both the pace of technological development and the fact that young people are in the vanguard of technology adoption make adult oversight difficult and even undesirable. In addition, it is unlikely that most adults will be able to provide support to young people to help them to deal with every negative piece of content that they experience on social media, given the huge volume of posts young people see and attend to. Instead, young people need to be equipped with the skills and qualities they require to engage with digital/online media safely.

A key quality that becomes evident from the narrative is resilience. Young people need to be able to 'bounce back' from the constant and unfettered exposure to images, photos, and videos of their peers' bodies and the impact these can have on levels of body dissatisfaction. To support the development of resilience, empathy is important. As identified in the dialogue between Chloe and Leah, some young people need a deeper understanding of the reasons why some people post 'perfect pictures' and why others may not. Equally, young people need to be supported to celebrate diversity and not reject it.

In the narrative, Chloe was empathetic to the skinny girls because she could relate to their body shape and size. Chloe had resilience in this context because she was able to understand that the skinny girls' posts were a potential reflection of their lower levels of self-esteem and that the skinny girls used social media as a resource to strengthen their positive feelings of self. On the other hand, Leah was critical of the skinny girls. She interpreted the skinny girls' posts as a somewhat selfish activity that was undertaken to make other young people her age feel bad about their bodies. Leah's critical actions exemplify the need to support young people to be more empathetic as a way of building resilience and to help young people to deal with the unfettered exposure to pictures, images, and videos of their peers' bodies.

Considerations

Social media is a powerful educational resource

Social media has the potential to be a *powerful educational resource* to support young people's development. With appropriate support, young people's exposure to the vast amounts of information available about health, and specifically the body, can be used to build resilience and develop empathetic understanding. Schools/teachers and parents/guardians should use this material, given its relevance in young people's lives and its impact on some young people's behaviours, cognitions, and emotions. Social media material can be used to open up dialogue about health and the body and to support young people's understandings of the reasons underpinning people's actions on social media and in wider society. In this sense, social media material can be used as an educational resource to build resilience and empathy, and has the potential to impact offline and online behaviours.

Peer-to-peer support is an important mechanism to support young people's uses of social media material

Peer-to-peer support is vital. Peers are highly influential in young people's lives. Clearly, young people can learn from peers and listen and respond to each other's actions. In terms of social media, young people have a greater contextual understanding of social media environments than adults, as well as an appreciation of the ways in which social media is used and the meanings ascribed to different social media material. Adults should appreciate the power of peer support and accept that young people will often turn to their peers instead of their teachers and/or parents/guardians. Young people often regard adults as

Table 4.1 Key messages about peer content

Characteristics of Young People's Uses of Social Media for Health	Young people view content posted and shared by their peers on social media. Images of the body posted by peers can, for some young people, act as a form of peer pressure, and encourage young people to think that they should change their health-related behaviours to look a certain way. Some young people do not experience peer pressure, as they understand or are able to make judgements on the potential reasons why some of their peers or other young people their age post particular content to social media.
Stakeholder Response Focused on Young People's Uses of Social Media for Health	Young people's constant exposure to images shared by peers of their bodies encourages peer comparison and this can lead to heightened levels of body dissatisfaction. Comparing oneself to others who are of the same age, gender, and from a similar context or school is extremely powerful and may not be helpful for some young people in constructing nuanced understandings about how to be a healthy young person. Resilience to such risks should be developed through supporting young people to be empathetic of the material posted by peers and through the celebration of diversity.
Considerations for Research, Policy, and/or Practice	Social media is a powerful educational resource. Peer-to-peer support is an important mechanism to support young people's uses of health-related social media.

unapproachable for discussions about social media because they lack the know-ledge and skills that young people would respect. As a way of better supporting young people to use social media safely and critically, adults need to provide pathways for young people to access peer support. In schools, vertical tutoring systems could be an option and/or the use of social media representatives. At home, dialogue between siblings about social media should be supported.

Section Three: key messages from the case

This case suggests that peer content (such as selfies) has a powerful influence on young people's levels of body satisfaction. It has also been suggested that social media is a powerful educational resource that can open up dialogue about the body. Resilience can be developed by supporting young people to engage with peer content and by encouraging peers to offer support and critical insights.

Note

1 The digital animated case study narrative video of Leah can be accessed here: http://epapers.bham.ac.uk/3061/

5 James

Likes

Victoria A. Goodyear, Hannah Wood,
and Kathleen M. Armour

Chapter overview

This chapter introduces, illustrates, and analyses the finding that 'likes' act as a form of endorsement and/or affirmation on the health-related information young people access and use on social media. 'Likes' mobilise health-related information and have a powerful influence on young people's health-related knowledge and behaviours. This chapter argues that adults need to better understand the complex ways in which health-related content is mobilised on social media in order to be able to offer support that will be effective. Social media surgeries are key spaces where adults and young people can learn about responsible social media use.

A digitally animated case study video of the evidence presented in this chapter can be accessed from: http://epapers.bham.ac.uk/3060/

Chapter structure and underpinning evidence

This chapter is organised into three main sections. In Section One a narrative of a young person – James – is presented to tell the story, from young people's perspectives, of how likes act as a form of endorsement and/or affirmation. The narrative was constructed from an extensive data set (as detailed in Chapter 1) and illustrates the voices and experiences of over 1,300 young people in the UK. Direct quotes from the data are shown in quotation marks. In Section Two – the stakeholder response – an interpretation of the narrative and recommended actions for research, policy, and practice are provided. The profile of the stakeholder group was international, multi-sector, and multi-disciplinary and included teachers, international academics (UK, Ireland, Sweden, Netherlands, Spain, Australia, China), and trusts/organisations in the UK (such as the NHS, Youth Sport Trust) that have a focus on youth health and wellbeing. The stakeholder group watched a digital animated video of the case study narrative[1] and collaborated to produce the response during a one-day workshop (as detailed in Chapter 1). In Section Three, the key messages that emerge from the narrative and the stakeholder response are summarised.

Section One: young person's narrative – James

'Feeling popular' on Instagram and Snapchat is really important to James. He says 'it feels nice to get a good amount of likes on your picture' and to have a 'high number of followers'. The way James talks about likes suggests that they act as a form of peer endorsement. James says that getting a like means a person literally 'likes' your post. In addition to likes, followers are also important and act as another form of peer endorsement. James says that having a high number of followers mean that people are interested in what you post to social media. **Likes and followers** *act as a form of endorsement and gaining likes and followers makes James* **feel good** *about himself.*

To find out whether he has any new *likes* or *followers*, James is on Instagram 'all the time'. 'After every hour he'll check Snapchat'. James checks his account 'every time he gets a notification'. He'll 'check it even if he doesn't have a notification', because sometimes there's a message and it doesn't tell you – it can be 'glitched'. So, James is tethered to social media. He is on Snapchat and Instagram before school, during school, and after school. Likes and followers are important to *James so he* **constantly checks** *Instagram and Snapchat for notifications of* **new likes or followers**.

James' engagement with social media for health

James has recently started to have 'competition type things' with his friends. The competitions are focused on 'who can get the most' likes or followers. So he bases his posts on what he 'thinks people would like to see', rather than 'what he likes'. He says that to get a high number of likes and followers he has to ensure that his posts 'please the fans'. So James took a 'nice-looking selfie' the other day, as apparently these get the most likes. He thought about taking 'a group photo' but these always seem to get 'liked less'. *Likes can be part of peer competitions and James has started to* **post nice-looking selfies** *to get* **more likes or followers than his friends**.

The 'like' competition has started to get a bit serious. James' mates stepped it up a level. They keep posting pictures and they 'like it themselves'. They also 'beg for them', saying 'like my recent post and I'll like it back'. Sometimes they even 'buy an app' to get likes from a random generator, so they are not even from real people. He also found out that 'most people make an account and then when their followers are getting active, they make another one to get all the other active followers to follow them, and they just keep making new accounts'. *James' friends* **tactically manipulate** *the* **functions** *of* **social media** *to get the most likes or followers.*

James didn't want to lose the 'competition', but he didn't want to beg for likes. He also couldn't afford the app. So he has started liking other people's pictures at school, even though liking their posts was a bit 'fake' and he was just 'laughing at' some of them. But liking other people's posts is also a 'risk'. James worries when people don't 'like you back'. He says that they might look at your posts and not 'like you back because you might not be as skinny as they want you to be', 'but you don't actually know'. *James started employing **different tactics** to his friends to get the most likes and followers, **even though tactics he used were a risk** as to how he feels about himself.*

James' tactics of liking other people's posts all went a bit wrong. James liked a picture of a girl at school. She had been 'really fat' but had 'lost loads of weight'. James thought she looked really good. But people had started commenting that she had 'taken it too far' and they started 'skinny shaming her'. When James liked her post he didn't realise that this would be interpreted as him re-enforcing her 'weight loss'. He also didn't realise that by liking it 'someone else could see it' with all the comments. Now more people could see it, and they were all 'laughing at' her. He didn't mean to do this, he just wanted to win the competition. He also didn't realise that she was in a state of 'depression' because of all the comments that were 'skinny shaming her'. James has seen people post about 'taking a break' from 'social media because they're depressed'. He has also heard about people becoming 'suicidal' because of body comparisons on social media. But he had never thought that his 'competition' could cause anyone any harm. *The **tactics** James used to get the most likes and followers could result in **harm** for other people's **physical and emotional wellbeing**.*

People perceive things in different ways on social media. Some 'people get offended by something that someone else won't find offensive'. 'Context is quite hard', you just 'don't know how other people will feel'. Some people will post 'to see what people think of you'; for others, it's just a game. For James, his game turned out badly. *The way James used social media was **focused on himself** and this behaviour had **negative consequences** for other people's health and wellbeing.*

Narrative summary

Likes and followers act as a form of endorsement and gaining likes and followers makes James feel good about himself. Likes and followers are important to James, so he **constantly checks** Instagram and Snapchat for notifications on **new likes or followers**. Likes can be part of peer competitions and James has started to **post nice-looking selfies** to **get more likes and followers than his friends**. James' friends tactically manipulate the functions of social media to get the most likes or followers. James started employing different tactics to his friends to get the most likes and followers, even though the **tactics he used were a risk for how he feels about himself**. The tactics James used to get the most likes and followers **could result in harm** for other people's **physical and emotional wellbeing**. The way James used social media was **focused on himself** and this behaviour had **negative consequences for other people's health and wellbeing**.

Section Two: stakeholder response

Young people can become addicted to gaining likes and followers. On the one hand, young people can become addicted to social media itself and the access to constant social interaction. On the other hand, young people can become addicted to feelings of being popular. In this respect, social media is a powerful resource that can be used to support young people's social and emotional needs. The theoretical framework of social capital can be helpful in explaining how social media is a resource; for example, social media can be considered as a currency which young people use. To support young people, adults need to better understand the complex ways in which young people use social media and how they manipulate the functions of social media. Youth-centric understandings of social media will enable adults to offer appropriate support. Social media surgeries and local health and wellbeing organisations are important spaces in which young people and adults could learn more about the interactive functionalities of social media and the related impacts.

Addiction

One reading of James' behaviour is that he is addicted to social media. James constantly checks his social media accounts and is permanently tethered to his mobile device. Given that time spent on social media is strongly associated with mental health challenges, the way in which James is using social media is concerning. The time he is investing in being on social media has the potential to lead to symptoms of stress, anxiety, and depression.

Another reading of the narrative is that James is addicted to feelings of being popular. James appears to be fixated on gaining attention through social media via likes. In many respects, ensuring that he gains a high number of likes has become a habitual behaviour and offers an explanation as to why James was not aware of how his actions could result in harm for others. It was also evident that James' friends were buying likes, and this appeared to be a compulsive act to fulfil their needs to feel popular. The way James and his friends used social media could therefore be interpreted as a symptom of an underlying social or emotional problem. Although extreme, James' behaviour could be likened to the understanding that acts of criminality are often associated with underlying problems related to – for example – drug addiction.

Both of the readings of James' behaviour suggest that he is using social media to support his social and emotional wellbeing. Social media is a space for him to socially interact and 'likes' act as a pathway for James to feel socially accepted. Questions, however, must be raised in relation to James' offline social support networks. The extreme ways in which James uses social media suggests that he requires social media to fulfil other needs that are not being met offline. To support James, further evidence is required about his social and emotional wellbeing. The narrative provides an outsider's view of James' uses of social media, and researchers, schools/teachers, and parents/guardians need to be cautious about making assumptions about young people's health and wellbeing based solely on evidence about how young people use social media.

Social capital

The ways in which young people use and manipulate likes and followers is an example of building and deploying social capital. Through likes and followers, young people have created a currency within which to position themselves within a vast social network. Likes and followers, in this sense, act as a social and emotional resource for young people.

Young people's awareness of how to capitalise on social media to attract attention and gain influence should be respected. Through participating in social media, young people have learned key components of advertising literacy and marketing strategies. James, for example, learnt of the types of posts that are required to attract attention. He also learnt of the importance of interacting with others in order to gain influence. These are key skills relevant to society, and social media was helping James to learn how to engage with public audiences and in public spaces. In one sense, it could be argued that James was employing a sound marketing strategy.

Despite social media providing opportunities for broadening young people's social networks (as also seen in Chapter 2), there are two key issues of concern related to social capital and James' behaviour. First, it could be argued that young people are manufacturing their wellbeing through social media and this can have negative consequences. The currency of likes does not adequately replace the interpersonal nature of interaction, with followers and likes failing to replace the characteristics of friendship or belonging to a social group. As stated by James, likes were also fake and could be illustrative of ridicule rather than social support. The second issue relates to the content young people are creating to gain likes or followers. Given that 'polished', 'perfect', and 'idolised' posts have a powerful influence over young people's wellbeing (as seen in Chapter 4), young people may not be acting in ways that are socially responsible. By going to extreme measures to gain likes, as was evident in James' behaviour, the content of posts could attract unwanted attention. If posts are driven by the desire for affirmation and are used as a tool for social positioning, young people become vulnerable to self-doubt, potentially leading to the development of lower levels of self-worth and self-esteem.

Considerations

Young people should be treated as 'expert' users of social media and their experiences and opinions should be sought to help adults better understand the complex ways in which social media is used

There is an urgent need to develop youth-centric understandings of the ways in which young people use social media. Currently, parents/guardians lack the understandings they require to engage effectively in the digital/online environments inhabited by young people, and they also lack the digital skills required to engage with, navigate, and appreciate digital youth culture. Schools/teachers and parents/guardians, therefore, require a much more detailed understanding of the ways in which young people use social media, the nature of any impacts on health and wellbeing, and evidence-based examples of good practice. Young people's own discourses of risk and their perspectives on how they negotiate and navigate digital environments can provide schools/teachers and parents/ guardians with deeper understandings of digital spaces and cultures that are often far removed from adult experiences.

Support needs to be provided by local organisations and social media companies

Local health and wellbeing organisations and social media companies are well placed help young people to learn how to use social media responsibly, and to empower them to engage with the potentially positive opportunities of digital media for their health and wellbeing. Social media surgeries are useful spaces in which young people and adults can gain support on how to navigate social media and how to act responsibly online. Social media companies, such as YouTube, are increasingly leading workshops to support safe and ethical social media practice. Local health and wellbeing organisations are also an important space for young people to access social and emotional support. Adults need to increase young people's awareness of these forms of support in order to encourage socially responsible behaviour and young people's wellbeing.

Section Three: key messages from the case

This case has illustrated that likes act as a form of endorsement and/or affirmation on the health-related information young people access and use on social media. The case suggests that adults require a better understanding of the complex ways in which health-related content is mobilised on social media, in order to be able to offer support to young people that will be effective. Social media surgeries and local health and wellbeing organisations are spaces where adults and young people can learn about the different ways in which social media can be used. A summary of the key messages of the case can be found in Table 5.1.

Table 5.1 Key messages about likes

Characteristics of Young People's Uses of Social Media for Health	A high number of likes or followers can make some young people feel good about themselves. Some young people carefully select the type of content that they post to ensure that they receive a high number of likes. Some young people also tactically manipulate the functions of social media to get the most likes or followers. This behaviour is highly self-focused. This self-focused behaviour and the tactics that young people use to get a high number of likes and followers can result in harm for other people's physical and emotional wellbeing.
Stakeholder Response Focused on Young People's Uses of Social Media for Health	Young people display addictive behaviours in terms of interactions and becoming 'popular'. Some media is a powerful resource that meets these needs. Social media can therefore play a positive role in young people's health and wellbeing. However, if young people have poor social networks, the addictive behaviour can have further negative impacts on their wellbeing. Social media relationships based on likes insufficiently replaces the characteristics of offline feelings of friendships and belonging.
Considerations for Research, Policy, and/or Practice	Young people should be treated as 'expert' users of social media and their experiences and opinions should be sought to help adults better understand the complex ways in which social media is used.
	Support needs to be provided by local organisations and social media companies.

Note

1 The digital animated case study narrative video of James can be accessed here: http://epapers.bham.ac.uk/3060/

6 Jess

Reputable content

*Victoria A. Goodyear, Hannah Wood,
and Kathleen M. Armour*

Chapter overview

This chapter introduces, illustrates, and analyses the finding that young people follow, share, and use health-related information that is shared by reputable social media accounts. The powerful influence of social media on young people's health-related behaviours suggests that social media should be harnessed by governments, health and wellbeing organisations, and schools/teachers as an important space in which to educate young people about their health. Yet, these stakeholders, as well as celebrities, sportsmen and -women, and 'sports' brands need to be aware of the trust young people place in them, and ensure that they too act responsibly on social media.

A digitally animated case study video of the evidence presented in this chapter can be accessed from: http://epapers.bham.ac.uk/3059/

Chapter structure and underpinning evidence

This chapter is organised into three main sections. In Section One a narrative of a young person – Jess – is presented to tell the story from young people's perspectives of how young people follow, share, and use health-related information that is shared by reputable social media accounts. The narrative was constructed from an extensive data set (as detailed in Chapter 1) and illustrates the voices and experiences of over 1,300 young people in the UK. Direct quotes from the data are shown in quotation marks. In Section Two – the stakeholder response – an interpretation of the narrative and recommended actions for research, policy, and practice are provided. The profile of the stakeholder group was international, multi-sector, and multi-disciplinary and included teachers, international academics (UK, Ireland, Sweden, Netherlands, Spain, Australia, China), and trusts/organisations in the UK (such as the NHS, Youth Sport Trust) that have a focus on youth health and wellbeing. The stakeholder group watched a digital animated video of the case study narrative[1] and collaborated to produce the response during a one-day workshop (as detailed in Chapter 1). In Section Three, the key messages that emerge from the narrative and the stakeholder response are summarised.

Section One: young person's narrative – Jess

Jess uses social media to follow 'celebrities' and to 'see the gossip'. Sometimes the 'celebrities' are 'sportspeople' or 'rappers'. Most of the time, however, Jess follows the stars of 'reality TV shows'; the ones that people call 'fake celebrities'. On social media, Jess can 'learn about their life', and she has seen them 'go from what they were to what they are now'. The 'fake celebrities' lives give Jess hope that she could become a celebrity one day. Jess is also inspired by 'something called the Instagram model'. The 'Instagram model' is where 'someone can be *so* famous' and 'only through a few pictures'. The 'Instagram model' is definitely something Jess could use. She just needs to post really 'polished' and 'perfect' images about her life and make sure that these posts get a lot of 'likes'. *Jess looks at **fake celebrities** on social media. She is inspired by the 'Instagram model' and the possibilities of becoming famous through a few pictures.*

Jess follows the 'fake celebrities' on Snapchat and Instagram. After all, these are the most popular social media sites at the moment. But while the 'fake celebrities' post 'perfect images' to both Snapchat and Instagram, young people Jess' age use Snapchat and Instagram differently. Snapchat is for 'funny stories', 'dog filters', and 'ugly pictures with double chins'. Instagram, on the other hand, is for 'perfect images'. Jess says that Instagram is 'your space to express yourself', it's like your 'little platform'. She says that you can 'photoshop' your pictures and this can help you to look a bit like the 'fake celebrities'. *Jess can use Instagram to **post perfect images** that are **photoshopped** and look a bit like the **fake celebrities*** she follows.

Jess' engagement with social media for health

Jess is 'tired'. She stayed up until '1 a.m. going through her [social media] feed', and she had to get up at '6:30' for school. This is typical for Jess. But last night 'everyone' was up late. 'BB', the latest teen celebrity, had an Instaspree (posting lots of posts in a short period of time) and everyone was Snapchatting about BB's posts. BB is one of the 'fake celebrities'. 'Most of her isn't real'. Everyone knows it's all 'money and surgery'. BB always tries to fake it though. She adds hashtags like #fit #gym #hardwork to try to trick everyone into believing that her figure has been developed through exercise. Yet, even though everyone knows BB is 'fake', girls like Jess 'still want to grow up to be like' her. *Teen celebs try to **trick users** of social media to think their figures are **real** and are a **result of exercise**. Girls like Jess look up to these 'fake celebrities' and **want to be like them**.*

Sarah, Jess' friend, sent a Snapchat being all jealous of BB, 'oh, I wish I looked like her'. Sarah was keen to find a way to look like BB. She later Snapchatted: 'I've seen on social media one of these waist trainers. My Mum said if you want one you can get one, I'll pay half you pay half'. Jess wasn't sure about the waist trainer, and sent a Snapchat, saying that it 'crushes your ribs'. Jess didn't want to use the waist trainer like Sarah, but she did want to look like BB. *On social media, girls learn about **harmful devices** that they can use to **change*** *their shape and figure. Jess is critical of these devices and she **knows** that the use of some these devices **can result in harm**.*

Jess wanted to find other ways to help her look like BB, a way that kept her ribs intact. So Jess scrolled through her Instagram home page. She found images and videos that said: 'Eating 10 kilograms of protein will help you build muscle every day'; 'The benefits of a hot and cold shower'; 'Sleep on your left side' to benefit 'your heart'; 'Smoothie that … gets rid of the bacteria on your face … and gives you *so* much energy'. Jess was bombarded with these health 'short-cuts', all of which she could use. But Jess found it difficult to determine what would work and what wouldn't. She is aware that information on social media is 'not always true'. There is 'no filter' and sometimes it can 'be just a scam'. It's like Trump's fake news, '#runfromTrump'. In addition to this, although young people Jess' age trust social media posts made by the government, health, and wellbeing organisations and sports men and women, the posts made by these reputable accounts often share the same types of information that Jess knows to be 'fake' or harmful. *Jess was bombarded with **information** on social media about how she can **change her shape and figure**. Jess found it **difficult** to work out **what information was credible and legitimate**.*

Jess decided that her only option was 'Photoshop'. Photoshop was something she could trust and control. She could take 'a picture and edit it and actually look great'. Jess knows that this is what all the 'celebrities' and 'models' really do. So Jess spent two hours, in between Snapchatting Sarah, trying to get something 'perfect' to post. But although Jess was Photoshopping her photo, she didn't want it to it to look fake. Sometimes 'you can just tell that they are fake', 'you can see that they've Photoshopped it'. Jess wanted the real kind of fake; something that would present the 'perfect image' of the 'real her'. ***Jess* decided to *Photoshop her pictures* to try to *look like the fake celebrities*. Photoshop meant that she could portray the *perfect image of the real her*.**

Jess posted the picture to Instagram. She immediately got loads of likes. By the time she woke up, she had 200 (which is good). The Photoshop had worked and she had 'faked it' well. To Jess' disappointment, however, she didn't get any comments. Comments are better than likes. BB always got loads of comments, and 'thousands, millions' of likes. Jess didn't understand what she was doing wrong. Try again she thought; try filters as well – the ones the celebs use. The filters that make you think, 'oh, that is me and I look the bomb'. Failing that, Jess said she'll have to copy Sarah and get a waist trainer. *Jess' picture received a **lot of likes but no comments**. This signalled to Jess that she needed to take **more extreme measures** to ensure her pictures received comments and likes. Jess considered the **use of the harmful devices** so she could look more like the fake celebrities.*

Narrative summary

Jess looks at **fake celebrities** on social media. She is inspired by the 'Instagram model' and the possibility of becoming famous through a few pictures. Jess can use Instagram to **post perfect images** that are **Photoshopped** and look a bit like the **fake celebrities**. Teen celebs try to **trick users** of social media that their figures are **real** and are a **result of exercise**. **Girls like Jess look up** to these 'fake celebrities' and **want to be like them**. On social media, young people learn about **harmful devices** that they can use to **change their shape and figure**. **Jess knows** that the use of these devices **can result in harm**. Yet, Jess is bombarded with **information** on social media about how she can **change her shape and figure**, and Jess finds it **difficult** to work out **what information is credible and legitimate**. Jess decided to **Photoshop her pictures** to try to **look like the fake celebrities**. Photoshop meant that she could portray the **perfect image of the real her**. Jess' picture received a **lot of likes but no comments**. This signalled to Jess that she needed to take **more extreme measures** to ensure her pictures received more comments and likes. Jess considered the **use of the harmful devices** so she could look more like the fake celebrities.

Section Two: stakeholder response

Social media acts as a strong force of ideological persuasion on the ways in which young people believe they should be healthy. Material posted by role models and the bombardment of available unhealthy products can cause a clear suspension of consciousness about how to be a healthy young person. Through modelling the behaviours of others on social media, health becomes a public performance and is associated with displaying a perfect body image. Yet, the powerful influence of social media on young people's health-related behaviours highlights that social media should be harnessed positively by governments, health and wellbeing organisations, and schools/teachers as an important space in which to educate young people about their health and wellbeing.

Reality

Young people are immersed in social media. The narrative shows that they are deeply engrossed in social media material shared by their 'role models' and that young people live their lives with, by, and through these distant and largely (personally) unknown individuals. The social media spaces in which young people participate in are also awash with unregulated and unsolicited health-related content, and young people are bombarded by unhealthy products. As Jess illustrates, the material accessed from role models, together with the barrage of unhealthy products, can act as a strong force of ideological persuasion about how to manage and present body image in order to be 'healthy'. In many respects, Jess was being hypnotised by the sheer volume of unhealthy messages in which she was immersed. There is evidence from the narrative to suggest a clear suspension of consciousness that, intensified through her lack of sleep, was causing Jess to exist in an 'open trance' where reality meant being 'unhealthy'. In using social media in a way similar to Jess, young people will be challenged to accept and adopt alternative health-related messages.

It is a concern that the narrative suggests that parents/guardians are doing little to help young people navigate the harmful messages in which they are immersed on social media. Instead, some parents/guardians are (unwittingly) supporting young people to be and become unhealthy. Although access to social media should be treated as a right, the regular use of social media until '1 a.m.' is harmful physiologically and will impact negatively on young people's social and emotional wellbeing. The need for parents to become more educated in order to help young people address such harmful behaviours is further illustrated by the actions of Sarah's mother. The offer of financial support to buy a waist trainer signals that Sarah's mother was unaware of the potential negative impacts of this device on Sarah's health. Equally, Sarah's mother was willing to accept that health-related information on social media would be credible. It is possible that Sarah's mum was trapped in the same 'open trance' state as Sarah.

Despite negative impacts seen in Jess, the underlying actions of ideological persuasion could be used for health promotion. A reality that portrays health as supported by being active, eating well and getting adequate sleep could be presented to young people through role models and increased exposure to 'healthy' information. In seeking out social media as a health promotion tool, the narrative highlights some key content, design, and interactive features of social media into which health educators could tap. In particular, governments, health and wellbeing organisations, and schools/teachers, as well as celebrities, sports men and women, and 'sports' brands need to be aware of the trust young people place in them, and ensure that they, themselves, act responsibly on social media.

Health as a public performance

Health in the narrative was an outward-facing activity. Instead of young people associating health with physical, social, and emotional feelings and behaviours, health was conceptualised by what could be displayed publically and shared on social media. In particular, a portrayal of a healthy body was associated with slenderness. The way in which Jess wanted to display her body on social media suggests that health was perceived to be a static entity that could be obtained, rather than being a dynamic state of multiple thoughts, emotions, and feelings. In turn, social media was useful to Jess because it meant she could control public perceptions of her health. The 'Instagram model' of health could be used to control the aspects of her body she wanted to share and emphasise with, while filters could be applied to ensure that her body conformed to particular idealised standards. Social media is therefore a space in which young people consume and reproduce unhealthy constructions of health in very public and highly visible spaces.

Considerations

Young people and adults require appropriate health education

To mitigate against the acceptance of narrow constructions of health, young people and adults require access to health education that extends beyond the material available on social media. There must be a concerted effort to support young people and adults to discern which types of health information are relevant and can be trusted. Educational activities should be structured through a critical pedagogy lens that allows young people and adults to inquire into their own social media behaviours and the information that is presented to them via social media platforms.

Social media should be harnessed by governments, health and wellbeing organisations, and schools/teachers as an important space in which to educate young people about their health and wellbeing

There are unprecedented opportunities to reach and engage with young people through social media given that social media use is a daily and almost continuous activity. Young people are constantly exposed to an influx of health-related messages, information is widely accessible, dissemination can occur quickly, and material that relates to young people can be easily retrieved. Young people also place a degree of trust in governments, health and wellbeing organisations, and schools/teachers, as well as role models that include celebrities and sports men and women. These stakeholders' uses of social media provide clear opportunities to engage large numbers of young people with health information that is credible and appropriate. Social media is, therefore, a relevant and engaging platform that provides opportunities to engage young people with appropriate information about their health.

Section Three: key messages from the case

This case has illustrated the ways in which young people follow, share, and use health-related information that is shared by reputable social media accounts. The powerful influence of social media on young people's health-related behaviours suggests that social media should be harnessed by governments, health and wellbeing organisations, and schools/teachers as an important space in which to educate young people about their health. Yet, these stakeholders, as well as celebrities, sports men and women and 'sports' brands need to be aware of the trust young people place in them, and ensure that they, too, act responsibly on social media.

Table 6.1 Key messages about reputable content

Characteristics of Young People's Uses of Social Media for Health	Young people follow, share, and use health-related information that is shared by reputable social media accounts. Reputable accounts include the accounts of governments, health and wellbeing organisations, and celebrities, sportsmen and -women and 'sports' brands. Yet, young people are bombarded with information on social media about how they can change their shapes and figures. Some young people find it difficult to work out what information is credible and legitimate.
Stakeholder Response Focused on Young People's Uses of Social Media for Health	Material posted by role models and the bombardment of unhealthy products can cause a clear suspension of consciousness about how to be a healthy young person. Some young people conceptualise health as what can be publically displayed and shared on social media rather than associating it with physical, social, and emotional feelings and behaviours.
	To address these issues, a reality that portrays health as being active, eating well, and getting adequate sleep could be presented to young people through reputable social media accounts to increase young people's exposure to 'healthy' information.
Considerations for Research, Policy, and/or Practice	Young people and adults require appropriate health education.
	Social media should be harnessed by governments, health and wellbeing organisations, and schools/teachers as an important space in which to educate young people about their health and wellbeing.

Note

1 The digital animated case study narrative video of Jess can be accessed here: http://epapers.bham.ac.uk/3059/

7 Young people's recommendations and actions for schools/teachers, parents/guardians, and social media companies

Victoria A. Goodyear, Hannah Wood, and Kathleen M. Armour

Chapter overview

This chapter introduces, illustrates, and analyses the finding that parent/ guardians and schools/ teachers are currently ill-equipped to support young people to make informed decisions about their engagement with health-related social media. Data shows that support from adults is welcomed by young people, but that adults require a better understanding of the complex and dynamic ways in which young people use social media. Peer-based support is also important, given young people's contextual knowledge about social media. The case suggests that adults and peers can help young people to choose how to respond to health-related information and how to determine credible information.

Chapter structure and underpinning evidence

This chapter is organised into three main sections. In Section One, a narrative is presented to tell the story of young people's frustrations with how adults interpret their uses of social media. The narrative was constructed from an extensive data set (as detailed in Chapter 1) and illustrates the voices and experiences of over 1,300 young people in the UK. The narrative is presented in the form of a WhatsApp conversation, that one group of young people selected as a relevant way of communicating their experiences of social media to adults. Direct quotes from the data are shown in quotation marks. In Section Two, an overview of how young people perceive they should be supported by adults to navigate and use health-related material on social media is provided. These recommendations and actions were constructed from 50 young people during a one-day workshop (as detailed in Chapter 1). The young people watched videos of the case study narratives presented in Chapters 2–6 and were asked to create a response for adults. Data were drawn from resources young people created such as radio or TV interview, podcast, video/movie, or a newspaper article. Direct quotes from the data are shown in quotation marks, and pseudonyms are used. Quotes are also used from the resources young people created and are referred to as artefacts. In Section Three, the key messages that emerge from the narrative and the workshop are summarised.

Section One: young people's narrative – Kelly, Yaz, Leah, James, and Jess

'Kelly', 'Yaz', 'Leah', 'James', and 'Jess' (from Chapters 2–6) were members of a WhatsApp group. Despite the group members having different experiences of health-related social media (see Table 7.1), they all used social media to interact with friends.

The WhatsApp group was named Pengting, a word used by young people to say that someone is attractive. One interpretation of the WhatsApp group's name is that the discussions on this social media site would all be about body image. From the name, it could be assumed that the group members are obsessed with their bodies being perfect. This perspective is, however, the adult understanding of the group name. The WhatsApp group members had named the group Pengting as a joke. Pengting is just one of the latest words young people use and is a throwaway term. Pengting is similar to terms such as 'sick' that means good not poorly; 'bare' that means really or lots of; and 'dench' that means the same

Table 7.1 The different ways in which Kelly, Yaz, Leah, James, and Jess experienced health-related social media

Kelly	Kelly uses social media to stay connected with her friends. She does not search for information about health and wellbeing on social media, but, through posts her friends like and automatically sourced accounts, Kelly sees large amounts of health and wellbeing-related content. Through using social media to stay connected with her friends, Kelly has learnt about many health-related workouts, diets, and products, including FitTea.
Yaz	Yaz uses social media to find quick and easy information that is relatable to him and relevant to his perceived needs. Yaz relates to the body transformation videos that he sees on social media as he wants to become more muscular. Yaz has started to act on the videos that he sees on social media, despite the videos being harmful for his physical development.
Leah	Leah uses social media to look at and share posts made by her friends. Young people Leah's age post pictures of their bodies on social media to get attention, but Leah is too self-conscious to post pictures of her body. Leah compares her body image to the pictures of her friends on social media and feels a level of peer pressure to look a certain way.
James	James is addicted to getting a high number of likes and followers from his posts to social media. To get a high number of likes and followers James posts selfies and engages with competitions focused on who can get the most likes and followers. His behaviour on social media is very self-focused and the tactics James used to win the 'likes' competition negatively impacted on another girl's wellbeing at his school.
Jess	Jess admires 'fake celebrities' on social media and wants to look like them. On social media, Jess is bombarded with information about how she can change her body image to look like the 'fake celebrities'. Jess finds it difficult to determine what information is legitimate. Jess used Photoshop to try and create the perfect picture but considered using a waist trainer instead when her post didn't receive enough comments.

as sick and is used to identify something as good. The problem the members of the WhatsApp group experience, like many other young people their age, is that adults don't really understand the language they use to communicate and the ways in which they use social media. There is an overwhelming tendency in adults to assume the worst and because they don't understand social media, almost every word or post is perceived as a risk.

This narrative tells the story of the Pengting WhatsApp group's frustrations with adults' limited understandings of the ways in which they use social media. The narrative is told through the Pengting group's WhatsApp messages to reflect one of the ways in which the young people wanted to communicate their message and because this form of dialogue also reflects the contemporary ways in which young people interact with each other.

The WhatsApp messages

The messages on WhatsApp were in response to recent events at school about social media and health. It had been announced in the previous week by the Pengting group's Head of Year that there would be an assembly on social media. This assembly was the third that term on the same topic. This time, however, the assembly was going to be about social media and health. One of the girls at school had started to suffer from anorexia because of something she had seen on social media and so the headteacher had initiated assemblies for all year groups.

'Ping!' Kelly's (see Table 7.1) WhatsApp alert went off ... and again ... and again. She looked at her phone and had loads of unread messages in the 'Pengting' group. Leah (see Table 7.1) had sent a series of messages and she clearly wanted to vent about the social media and health assembly tomorrow. Leah was frustrated by the teachers' assumptions that, because one person had a bad experience, everyone else could be affected in the same way. Leah was also worried that the teachers were reverting to their typical protection-orientated approach and would confiscate their phones.

17:53 LEAH: As if we have a social media and health assembly tomorrow just because that Anna girl in 10RJS got 'anorexia'

17:53 LEAH: I get that she 'got affected' by social media and that people were 'skinny shaming' and 'laughing at her'. That is bad, and yeah there are 'loads of risks' but not for everyone. Not for us!!!

17:54 LEAH: They will just use it as another reason try to ban us using phones! It is always the same when something bad happens

Kelly had forgotten about the social media assembly. The assemblies on social media were a running joke. The teachers always say the 'same thing', normally reminding them all to 'put their privacy settings up' or telling them about 'cyberbullying'. The teachers perceive that they are doing a good job of protecting young people from social media. The problem is, they 'don't really talk about' the important stuff. They don't talk about 'peer pressure' (as Leah had experienced see Table 7.1) on social media or all of the 'perfect bodies' with which everyone in the Pengting group are bombarded. These are the real risks of social media and the assemblies aren't, therefore, perceived as relevant.

18:01 KELLY: yeah and what are they going to even say!? It is not like 'a lot of the teachers here can really help!'

18:01 KELLY: 'I have Miss Williams' … 'I doubt she uses Snapchat everyday'

18:02 KELLY: They don't even know what we see on social media … or what we actually look at

18:02 JAMES: 👍

James 'liked' Kelly's messages. This wasn't a surprise to Kelly as James has a habit of 'liking' everything on social media (see Table 7.1). James was in agreement with Kelly. In the WhatsApp messages James sent, he started to ridicule the teachers for trying to talk to them about social media. The teachers didn't understand the way the Pengting group, like many other young people their age, interacted on social media. Teachers often misinterpreted their interactions and behaviours, particularly when they try to second-guess what emojis[1] mean. As a result, James felt that the assemblies were irrelevant to him and his uses of social media and he intended not to listen.

18:03 JAMES: Yeah 'I don't suppose they all know a lot about social media', especially the 'teachers who are more experienced' shall we say ☺

18:04 JAMES: It is pretty funny when they 'try to guess what emojis mean' and stuff though … obviously 'it's completely wrong!'

18.05 KELLY: Yeah and even though they don't have a clue, we are always getting 'lectures' from teachers saying 'Oh, do this, do that'. It's 'quite tiring'

18.06 JAMES: 👍

18:07 KELLY: 'PSHE is boring enough already!' They don't need to make assemblies even worse

18:07 LEAH: I bet they think that because we're all on social media this one is going to be really interesting, something we'll like

18:08 JAMES: I'm just going to try and stick my headphones in tomorrow. Don't think I'll be missing out on anything that is relevant to me

Yaz (see Table 7.1) joined the WhatsApp conversation. Yaz offered a different perspective to Kelly, Leah, and James. Yaz suggested that the social media assembly was an opportunity for everyone in their school to get the same information about social media and, in turn, reduce risk-related impacts. Assemblies, he felt, could reduce the number of people suffering from anorexia because information would reach everyone. Yaz also considered that his physical education teachers could be an important source of information and social support. In physical education, teachers could guide young people to the correct workouts to use for their age and to promote health.

18:10 YAZ: I would rather have a 'thing at school'! At least then 'everyone gets fed the same information' and there is more chance that less ppl will become anorexic coz of social media

18.11 KELLY: I completely disagree. I hate social media assemblies

18:13 YAZ: Yeah and I know you hate the assemblies Kelly … but I reckon some of the 'younger teachers in the school' could be pretty helpful

18.14 KELLY: like who?

18:16 YAZ: 'any of our PE teachers' could be pretty good at 'making sure that people know that they are able to go to someone to talk', 'if they are feeling inadequate'.

18:17 YAZ: like with workout videos, PE teachers could help us know 'which ones to watch and which ones to do'. Workouts which are 'age appropriate'

Although the Pengting group was frustrated by the assembly on social media and health, all group members agreed that they would prefer to be told about social media in school rather than at home and by their parents. Talking to parents, as can be seen from the WhatsApp messages below, was embarrassing and uncomfortable. Collectively, the group felt that their parents did not understand how they used social media. Parents' reactions were described as extreme and their responses were unhelpful. Parents would either ban their daughter/son from using social media or laugh at the uses of social media, with very little concern of risk or harm. The Pengting group felt that neither of these responses were helpful.

18:21 YAZ: Also, much better than having to talk to my parents about it!!!!

18:21 YAZ: Can you imagine 'telling your mum about what's happened on Instagram. I don't think that's a very comfortable position to be in!'

18:22 JESS: erm no!! That would be 'just awkward'.

18:23 LEAH: not comfortable at all!! And 'if we tell our parents they would probably just ban us from using social media'.

18:23 JESS: 'They love you but they're not really our age so they wouldn't understand'. Just look at how they use it! 'They are on Facebook' and post things like 'oh, I did a fun run today'!!! Imagine if we did that! Haha

18:24 LEAH: Yeah my mum is on Facebook all the time posting things like 'out for a drink with friends'.

18:24 LEAH: She sent me a friend request the other day. I'm not sure she realises that we don't go on Facebook in order to avoid parents!

18:27 JAMES: My mum 'just doesn't get it'. She doesn't understand seeing stuff like fitspiration posts can actually be 'damaging'!

18:28 JAMES: I showed them to mum and now 'every time she sees something on Facebook about somebody's fitspo or whatever, she laughs and then she shows it to me and says, "Look how funny this is"'.

As the WhatsApp conversation continued, most of the group agreed that teachers' and parents'/guardians' knowledge about how young people use social media needed to be enhanced. Adults needed to: understand the contemporary pressures in young people's lives; be aware of the varying risks young people are exposed to on social media; and know strategies for how young people manage and cope with pressures and risks on social media. The Pengting group felt that this type of knowledge would provide adults with a better understanding of what young people 'actually do' on social media and would strengthen adults' ability to offer support that is relevant and effective.

18:40 KELLY: But maybe our parents should be 'informed'. Maybe someone has to tell them about the 'problems of our generation'. They 'know you best' and are 'the ones who know what's good for you'

18:42 KELLY: I know that Anna getting anorexia doesn't happen to everyone on social media but if our parents are 'made aware of the risks', maybe they can 'check if we are struggling!' Maybe that would mean no more stupid assemblies, talking about everything in 'stark contrast to what we actually do'!

18:50 YAZ: Yeah maybe adults need to be educated to understand what young people deal with on social media.

James offered a different perspective. James stressed that social media companies have a role to play in supporting young people to deal with pressure and risk. Social media companies, James highlighted, could filter and restrict what people can see.

19:02 JAMES: Or maybe it's the 'social media themselves' that should be doing something!

19:03 JAMES: It is them who are 'letting people do this'. There should be 'age restrictions' for inappropriate material; they should 'limit' the stuff we can see.

19:04 JAMES: Why do people our age need to know about FitTea!?!

19:06 KELLY: That's true! Social media companies 'can't control what people put on social media, but they can give advisory points'

19:08 JESS: Anyway, can we stop talking about school now. This has gone on way to long

The conversation finished with Jess' desire to change the focus of the conversation. The next day, the Pengting group was due to have their assembly about social media and health. It was clear from the WhatsApp messages that the young people were not looking forward to this because they felt the content would be irrelevant and would not reflect how they use social media.

Narrative summary

Young people perceive that adults over-estimate the risks of social media and this is due to a lack of understanding of the medium and the very dynamic ways in which young people interact. The educational support young people receive in the form of school assemblies is often **deemed to be irrelevant and outdated**. Young people do not feel that teachers are currently well placed to provide educational advice about social media given that they often **do not occupy the same digital spaces** as young people. Despite this, some young people believe school is the **most appropriate** setting to receive social media support and that teachers have the **potential to aid young people's navigation of social media**. In contrast, young people often do **not feel comfortable** talking to their parents about the **risks of social media**. In order to support young people, **parents and teachers need to increase their awareness** of how young people use social media, the risks they face, and how these risks are navigated. Some young people believe that **social media companies** have a **responsibility to minimise the health-related risks** of using social media.

Section Two: young people's recommendations and actions for adults

To better understand how young people could be supported to participate in social media, the authors of this book hosted a one-day workshop with young people in June 2017. Fifty young people aged 13–16 from varying UK schools attended the workshop at the University of Birmingham (see Chapter 1). Young people worked in groups and watched videos of the case studies. Young people were then asked to construct artefacts that could act as a resource targeted at adults to inform them about how young people their age should be supported to use health-related social media. The young people could create different types of resources including a radio or TV interview, podcast, video/movie, or a newspaper article. Each group was also asked to decide on the main message of their constructed resource what category of adult they wanted to reach, that is, a policy maker, a health and wellbeing organisation, their head teacher, teachers, or their parents/guardians. The data highlighted two key recommendations and actions for adults.

Adults' understanding of the influence of social media on young people's health and wellbeing should be improved

Adults require a deeper understanding of how young people use and navigate health-related material on social media. This message was explicitly detailed in a number of the resources constructed by the young people. The resources aimed to increase adult awareness of the negative impacts of social media on young people's health.

The young people perceived that adults were not aware of the types of material young people saw daily and/or the influence of these images on their health and wellbeing. For example, the opening line of a constructed newspaper article stated, 'May your life be as perfect as you pretend it is on Facebook'. The constructed article, titled 'False perfections', was aimed to be an informative resource for parents and it focused on the need for parents to better understand the impact of filtered images on young people's perceptions of their body image. The article went on to highlight how much of the material accessed from social media can have negative impacts:

> As parents of today's youth, we need to be aware of the impacts the media can have on their health and wellbeing. Over 50% of young people believe that social media is a good source of health information; Yes, this can be proved by some aspects of what they see, yet plenty can be proved to be negatively impactful.
>
> (constructed newspaper article)

The young people perceived that adults tended to disregard the pressures they experienced in their lives. This was emphasised in another constructed newspaper article that encouraged adults to understand that social media has a powerful influence on health and wellbeing behaviours. The article also sought to educate adults as to why young people turn to social media for health-related information and highlighted that young people needed to be educated about how to make informed decisions about what health information to use or ignore.

> Teenagers are under the influence of social media; this brings many negative thoughts into their minds when they could be focusing on education. Their diets seem to be based on sugary food, however, they try to fix this by having pathetic, unhealthy, un-natural drinks, such as FitTea, which is promoted by many celebs on social media. People must start educating and helping the younger generation in becoming more healthy for their wellbeing.
>
> (constructed newspaper article)

The young people also stressed that adults need to be aware of how their own behaviours on social media impact young people. This was particularly evident in the case of celebrities and it was emphasised that celebrities need to consider the material they share. For example,

> celebs should understand that the things they promote are dangerous and can influence many.
>
> (constructed newspaper article)

Finally, the young people strongly resisted the tendency for adults to ban social media. The young people stressed that adults needed to understand that social media is a powerful learning resource and should be used to support their learning about health and wellbeing, as well as other subjects in school. For example:

> Any technological device should be allowed.... We could be able to research any information, to help us quickly and easily. It's an everyday

tactic. For example, in history you can find out information that happened in a century and now.... Using a device can help students learn and make them become more independent.

(constructed newspaper article)

Overall, the responses from young people strongly suggest that they would welcome adult support to help them navigate and use health-related social media. To do this, adults require a better understanding of: (i) the impacts of social media on young people's health and wellbeing; (ii) the types of material young people access from social media; (iii) the reasons why young people turn to social media for health information; and (iv) how social media can be an important learning resource. Adults, such as celebrities, must also understand their influence on young people through social media.

Young people need to be better informed about the health-related material available on social media

Young people considered that they required a better understanding about the health-related material that is available to them on social media in order to help them make more informed decisions about their health-related behaviours. Although adults could offer this guidance, information from young people their own age was also considered to be very important. The young people emphasised that peers were more appreciative of the pressures they experience in their lives and understood the complex ways in which youth navigate social media. In turn, a number of the constructed resources were targeted at young people, aiming to encourage them to be critical of the health-related material that they access from social media.

A key aim of some of the constructed resources was to communicate to other young people how they might be negatively impacted by the health-related information that is available on social media. A good example of this was from a video of a constructed interview, that was created by a group of young people, that aimed to highlight how a young person was demotivated by the material on body image that had been accessed from social media. The interview also emphasised it was important for schools to have an increased focus on peer pressure and body dissatisfaction.

INTERVIEWER: As a young person, has how you view yourself been changed by social media?

INTERVIEWEE: You are definitely influenced by what you see and read and I think that has changed my perception of myself, yeah …

INTERVIEWER: Do you think school should focus more on peer pressure and body dissatisfaction?

INTERVIEWEE: Yeah I do, I think that it's an unseen issue that has occurred from social media. You do view your body differently by what you see and you get peer pressure to do certain things by your friends but also companies online.

INTERVIEWER: What do you see more of on social media on body image, motivation or demotivation?

INTERVIEWEE: I think for me personally I see, for me anyway, demotivation. Because you will see like, I don't know, a really good model body, and you want that but you know you can't really get that.

INTERVIEWER: Like false hope?

INTERVIEWEE: Yeah it builds up your dream and stuff.

(video interview artefact)

In other constructed resources, the aim was to help young people determine what types of health-related information was credible and could be used to inform their health-related behaviours. In many of the newspaper articles, images were used to display what had been photoshopped or what information was credible. Quotes supporting the images also sought to encourage young people to be critical of the images on social media they accessed. For example, 'you don't have to be what you see' (constructed newspaper article).

The resources these young people felt should be targeted at young people also sought to provide direction and guidance on what they should do when they accessed a particular health-related post. It was emphasised that young people should block users, report users, tell somebody about their experience and/or be critical of information. One constructed video-based resource that was filmed in the format of a movie communicated these messages by using different scenarios. For example:

FEMALE: I'm going to post this on Instagram … filter, filter, filter. Ok, so let me see how many likes and comments I have

MALE: You're fat, you're ugly, you're stupid, you're hair looks terrible

FEMALE: What the hell is this!?!

NARRATOR: What happened there is that she wasn't very critical about who she was following so they were now bullying her. Always make sure that if this happens to you that you block them and report them and always tell somebody.

(constructed video artefact)

Overall, the resources constructed by young people strongly suggest that they need support to better understand the health-related information that is available on social media. Young people require an understanding of: (i) the potential negative impacts of health-related material; (ii) how to determine credible information; (iii) and how they should respond to health-related material if they experience any harm. This information should be provided to young people by young people, given their contextualised knowledge of social media.

Section Three: key messages from the case

This case has illustrated that parent/guardians and schools/teachers are currently ill-equipped to support young people to make informed decisions about their engagement with health-related social media. The case argues that adults and peers can help young people to determine how to respond to health-related information and how to determine credible health-related information that they can use.

Table 7.2 Key messages on young people's recommendations for adults

Key Characteristics of Young People's Uses of Social Media for Health	Young people believe that adults over-estimate the risks of social media. Young people do not feel that teachers are currently well placed to provide educational advice about social media given that they often do not occupy the same digital spaces as young people. Despite this, some young people believe school is the most appropriate setting to receive social media support given that it is a space that can reach all young people. School support is important as some young people do not feel comfortable talking to their parents about the risks of social media. Some young people believe that social media companies have a responsibility to control and limit what young people can see and access, and by offering advice to young people.
Young People's Recommendations and Actions for Adults in supporting their uses of social media	Adults' understanding of the influence of social media on young people's health must be improved. Adults require a better understanding of: (i) the impacts of social media on young people's health and wellbeing; (ii) the types of material young people access from social media; (iii) the reasons why young people turn to social media for health information; and (iv) how social media can be an important learning resource. Young people also need to better informed about the health-related material available on social media in order to make better, informed decisions about their health-related behaviours. Young people require an understanding of: (i) the potential negative impacts of health-related material; (ii) how to determine credible information; (iii) and how they should respond to health-related material if they experience any harm.

Note

1 Emojis are ideograms and smileys used in electronic messages and webpages.

Part II

Disciplinary analysis of young people's engagement with health-related social media

8 Social media as a health resource

A salutogenic perspective

Mikael Quennerstedt[1]

Chapter overview

This chapter explores the consequences of pathogenic notions of health in terms of a focus on risk and disease. A salutogenic perspective is an alternative way of discussing young people, social media, and health. In a salutogenic perspective, health resources are the main focus. A salutogenic perspective can help to identify new and diverse resources that young people draw upon to support their health development, such as social relations and/or critical awareness. As a consequence, this chapter highlights the pedagogical potential of social media and how it can educate about health as part of living a good life.

Health: a salutogenic perspective

This chapter will consider the interesting but potentially impossible question about what health is – or isn't. In scrutinising the relationship between social media, young people and health, an essential starting point is to ask ourselves the following questions: what do we mean by 'health'? And, how can we say anything about this issue if we are not making our assumptions about heath clear?

What health is, or can be, is closely related to how individuals and societal institutions conceive health. Historically, understandings about health have been influenced in different directions by philosophy, religion, moral norms, politics and science (Nordenfeldt 1987; Tengland 2007; Tones and Green 2004). On one hand, health has relied on science to define health and to tell us what is healthy. In this context, health is often viewed as the opposite of disease. On the other hand, health has been regarded as something utopian, representing an ideal condition or direction for how people 'ought' to live their lives (Quennerstedt 2008). In this vein, Wright and Burrows (2004, p. 216) argue that ' "health" is a term used in diverse ways, linked to particular value systems, world views and socio-political, economic and cultural contexts'.

Many notions of health start from a position of normality where health is equated to a human being's normal condition. The consequence in policy as well as in practice is then a focus on deviations from this normality. This is sometimes described as *pathogenic* (= origins of disease) perspectives of health (Antonovsky 1979, 1987; Quennerstedt 2008).

> If one is 'naturally' healthy, then all one has to do to stay that way is reduce the risk factors as much as possible ... [and] ... facilitate and encourage individuals to engage in wise, low risk behaviour.
>
> (Antonovsky 1996, p. 13)

These deviations (i.e. not health) have either been scientifically normative or morally normative. Scientifically normative often refers to medical science or psychoanalysis. Morally normative refers to 'correct' behaviour. Examples of behaviours that may be interpreted as correct are a male gender, heterosexuality, or normal body size, weight and shape. Health equalling normal and the forms of deviations can be understood in Figure 8.1.

Interestingly, what tends to happen is that our interest is turned towards the left side of the oval in Figure 8.1, since the question of what is normal is not something we need to cure, protect, or even investigate (curative health efforts). Some interest is also directed towards the line separating normal from not normal, so that we can detect and prevent people crossing the line (preventative health efforts).

In scientifically normative views, health becomes a condition understood as the absence of disease. In turn, health is understood as a goal – a static condition – achievable through avoiding diseases or risks of diseases (Quennerstedt 2010). In morally normative views of health, at least today, health becomes an attractive appearance and a fit, beautiful body. Deviations from the unattainable ideals in society are constituted as unhealthy, and in some cases even immoral (Gard and Wright 2001; Fitzpatrick and Tinning 2014; Leahy, O'Flynn, and Wright 2013).

Health can, however, be conceived of in different ways and can be seen as something more than simply not being diseased or being low risk. Alternatives

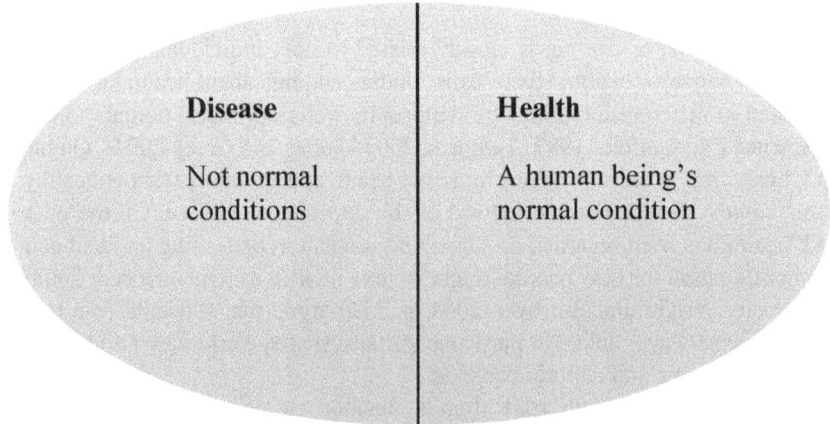

Figure 8.1 Health as the opposite of disease or not normal conditions.

to the pathogenic perspectives highlight the importance of psychological, social, societal, historical, and spiritual resources of health (Eriksson 2007; Lindström and Eriksson 2010). In the World Health Organisation [WHO] Ottawa charter, for example, this is formulated as: 'health is created and lived by people within the setting of their everyday life: where they learn, work, play and love' (WHO 1986, p. 2).

Alternative perspectives on health, that have emerged as a critique against the primarily biomedical notions of health, begin from a different philosophical standpoint to that of pathogenic perspectives. The perspectives can, as Antonovsky (1987) suggests, be termed *salutogenic* (= origins of health). The common denominator in a salutogenic perspective is a resistance towards health defined in a dualistic manner, as the opposite of disease or as not normal behaviour. Further, from a salutogenic perspective a critical stance toward the pervasiveness of pathogenic perspectives in research as well as in practice is taken (Lindström and Eriksson 2010; Mittelmark *et al.* 2017; Quennerstedt 2008). As Antonovsky (1979, p. 39) reminds us:

> Our linguistic apparatus, our common sense thinking, and our daily behaviour reflect this dichotomy. It is also the conceptual basis for the work of health care and disease care professionals and institutions in Western societies.

Health is accordingly not something you either have or do not have in salutogenic perspectives. Rather, it is about different degrees of health, on a continuum, created and sustained in an ongoing process (Lindström and Eriksson 2010) (see Figure 8.2). In this sense, everyone is in some way always healthy, and many aspects that promote or prevent health development can be encompassed. In a salutogenic perspective, diseases can of course affect people's health. Diseases are, however, regarded as separate processes that are applicable in certain situations as something that hinders health development, not as the opposite. Health is instead created in an interplay between the acting individual and her/his environment, so it is accordingly possible to have a disease and still be healthy.

In salutogenic perspectives, a large range of factors can promote or prevent health development on the continuum (Figure 8.2), for example, physical, social, political, spiritual, religious, economical resources, but also actions, diseases, and environmental factors. Antonovsky (1996) uses 'the river' as a metaphor to unpack these relational and sociocultural characteristics of health. As Antonovsky (1996, p. 14) states: '[w]e are all, always, in the dangerous river of life. The twin question is: How dangerous is our river? How well can we swim?'. How health is developed is then dependent on both our social, cultural, and

Less health  More health

Figure 8.2 Health as a continuum.

natural environment (the river), *and* the physical, social, and mental resources of the individual (how well we can swim) (Lindström and Eriksson 2010; McCuaig and Quennerstedt 2018). Addressing the twin questions of health, that Antonovsky reminds us of, makes salutogenic perspectives often focus on the presence of something positive like, for example, wellbeing, quality of life, democracy, equality, or meaningfulness. Health is further regarded as something dynamic, always in the process of becoming. So, returning to the initial question regarding what health is or isn't, the only answer we can provide is – it depends. However, what we should provide is an answer to what it depends on, and one such thing is our assumptions regarding health, and in consequence, what questions we ask regarding, in this case, young people, social media and health.

In scientifically normative (thus pathogenic) views of health, questions we tend to ask are related to risks connected to the use of social media. This includes questions about how social media enhances the risks for young people to develop eating disorders like anorexia or orthorexia, negative body image, depression, damaging social comparison, risky dieting, harmful self-objectification, wounding peer appearance-related feedback or increased body dissatisfaction. Social media is then toxic when it comes to health, and health is reduced to the absence of risk, disease, and not normal behaviour. As Antonovsky (1996) reminds us, efforts regarding health should logically then be focused on reducing these risks with social media and encouraging young people to engage in wise, low risk behaviour, such that a healthy use of social media becomes 'risk free'.

These risk questions and issues are unquestionably important when discussing young people, social media, and health. Society, education, and parents should of course protect young people and create stable structures regarding, for example, internet safety, restrictions on advertising directed at young people, parental control and/or educational efforts in school regarding risks related to social media. But is this everything regarding young people, social media, and health?

Before I return to this question in relation to the cases of young people presented in the book (Chapters 2–7), it is also important to say something generally about morally normative (thus pathogenic) views of health in relation to young people, social media, and health. It is important to note that scientifically normative perspectives are often amalgamated with moral norms with regards to health. Historically, homosexuality is an apt example which, at least in Sweden, was defined as a disease up until as late as 50 years ago. Here moral norms regarding sexuality are blended with a psychological allegedly scientific diagnosis (Lupton 2012; Rydström 2003).

Another example is body weight where scientific evidence of the medical risks of obesity is mixed with moral codes regarding overweight persons. Individuals measured as deviating from normal BMI (over weight = over normal BMI) are then categorised as being immoral, lazy, unhealthy, and are positioned as individuals who do not take responsibility for the societal economic project since they are constantly at risk of attracting costly diseases (Gard and Wright 2001). Burrows and Wright (2004, p. 193) argue that: 'Causal links drawn between ill health and moral laxity, sexual unattractiveness and emotional fragility have impelled even the most exercise-resistant of our population to action.' A beautiful, fit, and 'normal' body thus seems to be related to the value placed on us as human beings.

In morally normative views of health, questions we tend to ask regarding social media can be understood as related to young people's use of social media that is viewed as a behaviour deviating from the norm of adult behaviour. This is sometimes expressed as a moral panic over social media addiction, not dissimilar to how adults previously have fixated on computer games, video, television, and, historically, even reading novels. In this way, young people's social media use is positioned as the not normal and becomes hazardous and toxic per se, and as something adults and society should control and from which they should protect young people. In Chapter 7 this is captured beautifully by young people themselves. The chapter describes how young people interact in spaces that adults often don't understand or belong to, where 'every word or post is perceived as a risk' (p. 54).

At the same time, an interest concerning moral norms on health can help us scrutinise the amalgamation between scientific and moral norms. We can ask questions regarding how we can help young people to feel good about themselves despite strange body ideals that are prevalent in society in terms of muscular and thin, often commercially driven ideals. In relation to social media this can be about discussing what fitness is or isn't, and what norms the fitness industry drives young people to 'fit' into. We can also scrutinise moral norms regarding normal body weight and shape, individually measured as normal BMI, which are often promoted by societal institutions like education under the guise of saving young people from the 'obesity epidemic' (cf. Gard and Wright 2005; Harris *et al.* 2016; Petherick 2015; Powell and Fitzpatrick 2015). In this endeavour, it is important to be aware that well-meant campaigns about, for example, food also contain strong and persuasive moral norms regarding health.

Young people, social media, and health

When looking at the case studies in this book (Chapters 2–7) from a health perspective, that is, when the word health is used explicitly, it is quite easy to become dejected and even concerned. Health is depicted as a public performance of perfect bodies closely related to issues of diet, sleep, exercise, and body image. Social media then becomes a magnifying glass of society at large where slender and fit equals healthy, and overweight or fat (and sometimes even 'normal' weight) equals unhealthy (Fitzpatrick and Tinning 2014; Powell and Fitzpatrick 2015). In the chapters, health information, health-related material, dialogues about health, health literacy, and young people's health-related needs are mentioned, but with few clarifications regarding which information, what to have dialogues about, or what young people's needs actually are regarding health information and education. Jess' case (Chapter 6) is particularly powerful here because it indicates that what young people need regarding their understanding and development of health is ideologically persuasive messages about being active, eating well, and getting adequate sleep; messages that would preferably be delivered by celebrities. But this is, as I have argued, a quite narrow, individualistic, instrumental, and in many senses pathogenic notion of health.

Interestingly, the pathogenic description can also be the end of the story about young people, social media, and health when we look at it from a health perspective. However, what about WHO's (1986, p. 2) message that: 'health is created and lived by people within the setting of their everyday life: where they learn, work, play and love'? As I have argued earlier, in order to understand health, we also should ask salutogenic questions. In so doing, we have to take both the 'river' and 'the swimmer' into account, including both what promotes and hinders young people's development towards more health on the continuum (see Figure 8.2). So now let's put salutogenic questions to use in the cases provided in this book regarding young people, social media, and health.

Salutogenic questions can be posed in numerous of ways, capturing different aspects of the health continuum. In this chapter I use what Louise McCuaig and myself have developed in terms of identifying health resources through asking salutogenic questions (Ericson *et al.* 2017; McCuaig and Quennerstedt 2018). Briefly, health resources can be seen as different ways in which people from different backgrounds and in diverse contexts draw upon different resources to live a good life. As such, questions I would ask of the cases are:

- What does a good life for young people that involves social media look like?
- What hinders this good life?

Through posing these questions to the cases I have identified five health resources that young people draw upon in relation to social media:

1   Social relations, communication, and relatability
2   Education and learning
3   Public expression and affirmation
4   Knowing social media
5   Critical awareness.

Under each health resource I describe what promotes as well as hinders health development looking at the cases both regarding the 'river' and the 'swimmer'. Of course, a full account of the health resources can't be presented here, but it can illustrate a way to see how salutogenic questions help to explore and discuss issues of young people, social media, and health without reducing the conversation to risk alone.

Social relations, communication, and relatability

One important health resource regarding young people and social media is that social media can be a fantastic tool to communicate, contact friends, stay connected, and to talk to people instantly. This is visible in all the cases with Kelly,

Yaz, Leah, James, and Jess (Chapters 2–6) all conveying this clearly. Kelly (Chapter 2), for example, uses social media as a way to communicate with her friends, but also to connect to new people globally with shared interests to hers. In this way, she can with ease expand her social network beyond local social relationships and also, as seen in James' case (Chapter 5), generate social capital, even though James as reported in the case is capitalising the social in social media rather than creating social capital. Social media is also a way to relate to 'real people' through communicating with images and videos. Yaz (Chapter 3) describes this as helpful because both the information and the people communicating the information are relatable to him.

At the same time, the ease of the communication also makes it difficult to close down the communication, and this is sometimes referred to as a fear of missing out (FoMO) (Przybylski *et al.* 2013). Kelly (Chapter 2), in particular, describes this when she states that, 'if you haven't got Snapchat, it means you're a dead person'. It could be argued that this desire to always know what is going on with your friends can hinder health development. Also, James' case (Chapter 5) is an example where the ease of the communication on social media, together with the naivety of the user, magnify bullying and can make it more public in terms of, for example, fat-shaming or skinny-shaming that already occurs on social media.

Education and learning

Another important health resource in relation to social media is education and learning. In several of the cases social media is portrayed as a principal source of information. Social media thus becomes the instrument of learning in terms of knowledge about physical training from real people doing real exercises, as in Yaz's case (Chapter 3), or knowledge about people (celebrities or not) as in the case of Jess (Chapter 6). However, it is not only the information per se, but the opportunities to collaborate with and learn from others that become a powerful educational resource for dialogues about health. Indeed, Yaz (Chapter 3) suggests that social media campaigns can motivate people to be physically active. Through social media use, young people also develop the ability to communicate with images and videos, which can be seen as an important educational resource.

On the other hand, the cases also reveal that the social media sites young people use often portray an extremely narrow understanding of health, reducing health to a consumption practice and promoting health shortcuts. This can be devastating for young people's health development and, furthermore, the algorithms used in social media (see Chapter 2 and 3) seem to narrow the available information about health. The narrow notion of health portrayed on social media through its algorithms is a magnification of the media picture of health in society at large, and as a consequence we often position young people as vulnerable and in need of protection. This positioning of young people as vulnerable instead of competent can also be an obstacle for health development, and in Chapter 7 young people recommend that adults make an effort to understand contemporary pressures enhanced by social media and educate for an action competence in relation to the influence of social media.

Public expression and affirmation

The possibility of using social media as a space to express oneself publicly is something that can be seen as a health resource. This possibility to publicly express and post opinions and views through text, video, or pictures is more accessible and open for all on social media, and the cases show that the instant affirmation and endorsements in the form of likes, comments, and reposting, when posting something or sharing posts, can be fulfilling. James' narrative (Chapter 5) about feeling good about being noticed and getting positive peer feedback is interesting in this sense, since the endorsements on one hand seem to be part of James' idea of a good life, but on the other hand he can also reflect on the downsides that can make him feel bad about himself. Also, the WhatsApp group in Chapter 7 is powerful in the sense that it shows the deliberation of views and ideas in a 'publicly private' space where the young people can lash out at the not-knowing adults and get instant feedback.

At the same time, health through advertising and the sharing of pictures and videos can become a public performance associated with perfect bodies, where young people are looking for affirmation regarding their bodies. This, however, is not new, as health related to perfect bodies is an example of a morally norm-ative health perspective that was present pre social media (see Evans, Davies, and Wright 2004). It is, however, magnified through social media, and image filters creating images of perfect bodies, previously reserved for commercial media, are now available for everyone to use. Body dissatisfaction due to peer comparisons is thus potentially magnified, and as Leah's case (Chapter 4) high-lights, it is all more obvious when the peer comparisons are with people you know. Yaz's case (Chapter 3) is also interesting in terms of how he describes a rather narrow understanding of health, and Amy (his friend) expresses her con-cerns about health fanaticism connected to Yaz's physical training and focus on muscle-gaining exercises. At the same time Yaz highlights how physical activity campaigns can help with the motivation to be physically active if you see 'real people doing real exercises'.

Knowing social media

An important health resource in itself is the knowledge and ability the young people in the cases display regarding social media as a phenomenon. It is inter-esting to see how the cases display the ways in which young people are navig-ating social media; a medium where young people interact in spaces adults don't understand or belong to. The young people have specific knowledge about, in and through social media and ways to communicate with pictures and videos that most adults don't have. This knowledge creates a kind of meaningfulness and comprehensibility that is an important part of this health resource. In Chapter 7 the WhatsApp group is a fantastic illustration of how adults unsuccessfully try to grasp the complex ways young people use social media, and how this distinction of 'not being one of them' (i.e. the adult generation) becomes an important identity for a young social media user. It is 'us against them', it is 'us as knowers' and 'them as the not knowers' regarding an issue that is of actual importance. The young people pride themselves on being in a space and knowing it exhaustively in a way that adults (parents and teachers) are not even close to achieving, and this becomes an important health resource for them.

In Chapter 7, because of adults' lack of knowledge, school assemblies informing young people about social media became a running joke in the group, where adults talked about issues that were not important, for example, privacy settings. At the same time, adults failed to address issues that actually mattered to the young people, such as peer pressure. Leah (in Chapter 7) argued that because one person had a bad experience, adults then think that everyone is at risk, and James (in Chapter 7) claimed that adults are often completely wrong about what happens on social media.

The WhatsApp group discussions (Chapter 7) also highlight the need for social media navigational skills, that is, 'sailing without running aground'. The young people in the cases seem to be quite aware of the risks. They are already aware of the cyberbullying, the peer pressure, the focus on perfect bodies, the commercialism, and the fake images. What they seem to require is the navigational skills to navigate messages about health, to navigate the algorithmic properties of social media and the support to be able to withstand the pressures without the adults assuming the worst, because they don't understand social media.

Critical awareness

Another health resource closely related to the health resource of knowing social media (as above) that can be identified in the cases is critical awareness in relation to social media. This critical awareness is related both to being critically aware users and critically aware generators of social media. The Pengting WhatsApp group discussions (Chapter 7) and the advice young people give to parents, teachers, and other adults conveys the value of an inquiring critical stance toward the content in social media, but also towards social media in itself. The WhatsApp discussion (Chapter 7) demonstrates the ambiguity of this issue. Some of the young people think that school assemblies about social media are a waste of time, since adults don't know anything about what is going on in social media anyway. Yaz (in Chapter 7), on the other hand, thinks that assemblies can be an opportunity to get information out to all and reduce the risk-related impacts of, for example, anorexia. The young people also urge teachers and parents to increase their own critical awareness about what is happening on social media so that they can help young people to navigate against any potential risks. At the same time, none of them would ever talk about what is happening on social media with their parents and they mock adults' uses of social media, for example, the ways in which they use Facebook.

The cases also reveal that young people are, at the same time, aware and not aware users of social media. In a general sense, they are aware of the risks, and they also are aware of risks that adults don't know about. Amy's comments about Yaz's use of fitness videos in Chapter 3 is an example of this critical awareness. Also in the recommendations for adults (Chapter 7), this critical awareness is visible in that young people know they should block and report users who are cyberbullying, and that they should be critical of information on social media. However, this general awareness does not always extend to their own social media use. Amy (Chapter 3) is not critically scrutinising how social media campaigns affect herself, and Leah (Chapter 4) claims that 'there are loads of risks, but not for everyone. Not for us!!'.

Implications for addressing young people, social media, and health from a salutogenic perspective

From a pathogenic perspective, health is depicted as the opposite of disease or not normal behaviour. Asking pathogenic questions and considering the origins of disease in the cases thus involve issues of, for example, diet, sleep, exercise, and body image. However, it is seldom about good sleep, ample exercise, good eating habits, or positive body image. It is instead often about the risks involved in relation to these issues, and how we as adults should protect young people from these risks. As Antonovsky (1996, p. 13) reminds us: 'If one is "naturally" healthy, then all one has to do to stay that way is reduce the risk factors as much as possible … [and] … facilitate and encourage individuals to engage in wise, low risk behaviour.'

It is worth reminding ourselves at this point that pathogenic questions are important to ask, particularly in contexts of medicine. But just as risk, disease, or deviant behaviour become the answers to pathogenic questions, other issues *also* become important if we ask salutogenic questions, and this can occur without excluding risks. Risks instead become interesting if they hamper health development, but not as a risk in terms of deviating from a normal condition called health.

Looking at young people, social media, and health from a salutogenic perspective is accordingly not only about avoiding risks. Instead it is more complex than that, and the stories and experiences of over 1,500 young people in the UK illustrate the resources they draw upon in their social media use. This complexity is about developing and balancing resources for a good life, and the answers to salutogenic questions are related to origins of health, where sources for living a good life are found both in the 'river', with the 'swimmer', and in the relation between 'river' and the 'swimmer'. In this way, health can come in many different shapes and sizes: we might ask why we even attempt to talk about 'health' in the singular when we talk about so many different diseases. Is health rather a plural? Or is it even a noun? Is it something we do; that is, a verb: healthying?

Asking salutogenic questions accordingly makes us consider health resources such as social relations, education, public expression, and knowledge about social media, but the questions also reveal more aspects that can be barriers for health development beyond risks for disease. Examples of barriers for health in the cases are (i) not being on social media, (ii) the positioning of young people as vulnerable and adults always assuming the worst, (iii) peer comparisons, (iv) the algorithmic properties in social media, and (v) rampant commercialism targeting young people. But what can we do in school to encompass social media while taking health issues both in 'the river' and with the 'swimmer' into account? In the following, an example from Australia and a discussion about critical awareness and digital citizenship is presented to discuss some implications for education regarding young people, social media, and health from a salutogenic perspective and from the data presented in the case studies (Chapters 2–7).

The healthy-living website

One interesting example of what I have written so far is from Australia, where a salutogenic perspective of health is embedded in the national curriculum in health and physical education under the label of a strengths-based approach (Macdonald 2013; McCuaig, Quennerstedt, and Macdonald 2013). McCuaig, Quennerstedt, and Macdonald (2013) argued that the introduction of a salutogenic approach in the curriculum could potentially stimulate new opportunities regarding the learning area of health, where issues of social media form part of the curriculum. They illustrate this through a project – The Health Literacy @ Ipswich Schools project – where inquiry-based pedagogies were used in a salutogenically oriented health literacy unit of work. So, instead of teaching health literacy in health education as a pathogenic solution to issues such as sexually transmitted diseases, drug misuse or mental health, the unit explored a variety of life experiences and resources 'that support, inspire and promote young people's healthy living' (McCuaig, Quennerstedt, and Macdonald 2013, p. 117). An example of this is first a brainstorming session around the statement 'I am healthy and enjoy life because ...', and McCuaig, Quennerstedt, and Macdonald (2013, p. 117) write that:

> In response, students not only identified relatively pathogenically oriented concerns such as safe sexual activity and drinking, but also nominated learning to relax, owning a pet, quality sleep, positive friends and good communication with parents as focal themes.

The students also engaged in an assessment task that involved creating a healthy-living website for young people. On the website, the young people presented resources available to them among friends, in their family, in school and in their community, and related these resources to the needs of young people in Ipswich (McCuaig, Quennerstedt, and Macdonald 2013). In this task, social media could also have been scrutinised by young people in terms of questions like: 'I enjoy life because social media helps me to ...'. The adoption of salutogenic approaches in school practices have yet to be investigated, however, at state level the 'new' senior health education syllabus in Queensland for implementation in 2019 (Queensland Curriculum and Assessment Authority 2017) takes the salutogenic turn a step further, also including salutogenesis as subject matter and thus part of the assessment in health education.

Education, critical awareness and digital citizenship

When looking at the role of schooling in relation to social media in a salutogenic perspective, the cases in the book have implications for issues including education, critical awareness, and, in consequence, digital citizenship (Mossberger *et al.* 2007; Mossberger 2009). So how can we, in line with the 'Health Literacy @ Ipswich Schools project', educate young people to become 'healthy' users of social media? What can the role of education be regarding young people, social media, and health?

In the cases, and in particular in the advice young people gave to parents, teachers, and other adults (Chapter 7), it is argued that adults need to understand the contemporary pressures in young people's lives, as well as support young people to navigate risks related to social media. Critical skills and a critical awareness are in the cases highlighted as important, but what is being critical in this context, and what is it to act critically in a salutogenic perspective?

According to Johnson and Morris (2010), acting critically can be about critical thinking, which they argue is a rather individualistic and context-neutral way of looking at critique. On the other hand, Johnson and Morris (2010) also emphasise critical pedagogy as a collective, context-driven perspective which concerns equal opportunity and social justice. The two perspectives on critique sometimes intersect and if we take both of these aspects of critique into account, then teaching critical awareness and to act critically in relation to health can be several things.

First, it can be about teaching a critical stance not only towards social media itself, including social media algorithms or commercial interests on social media, but also towards messages about health in general. This might include messages promoting strange body ideals and measures such as BMI, pro-anorexia hashtags or extreme fitness videos. Second, the difficulty in teaching critical awareness is the question of what to be critical towards, and the cases highlight this difficulty and disparity between teachers' and young people's ideas regarding the focus of the critique. Education should then consider critical awareness in terms of *how* to be critical. In this endeavour, the question of *what* to be critical towards will inevitably change and will also be open for deliberation. So, what to develop a critical awareness about in school is a question of teaching more about *how* social media is used and practiced than *what* social media contains, since the content will constantly change. This is more about becoming members of a digital society, and Johnson and Morris (2010) in their discussion argue for critical citizenship education, and in the context of this chapter, I would add a digital citizenship education regarding health.

A salutogenic digital citizenship education could, as Lawy and Biesta (2006) argue, build on an inclusive and relational view of citizenship-as-practice. This perspective aligns well with a salutogenic perspective of health and the metaphor of the swimmer in the river. This involves a pedagogy *with* rather than *on* young people focusing on issues important to the young themselves. As Henry Giroux (2003, p. 12) argues: 'educational work needs to respond to the dilemmas of the outside world by focusing on how young people make sense of their experiences and possibilities for decision-making within the structures of everyday life'. It is accordingly not about guiding young people towards a pre-defined goal about what health is or isn't as established by society, education, or adults. It isn't either only about teaching young people about risks with social media as identified by adults. Instead it could be about a pluralistic and participatory social media pedagogy where young people can critically examine values, norms, and knowledge on social media in order to form their own nuanced standpoints. In this sense, as Andersson and Öhman (2017) argue, social media can be considered as a public pedagogy and young people's engagement in social media thus has clear educative potential. In turn, salutogenic digital citizenship education could focus on *how* social media is practiced in relation to health in a wider sense.

If we follow Giroux's (2003) advice to education, that it has to respond to the dilemmas of the young, we should let young people examine and discuss social media in a wide sense regarding health both as resources and as barriers for living a good life. Digital citizenship in relation to health is then about how to live a good life in different ways in a society where digital issues are a major part of people's lives.

Summary of key messages

From a salutogenic perspective on health:

- We have to look for origins of health both in terms of health resources and what hinders health development if we want to understand issues of young people, social media, and health. Health resources can then be understood as different ways in which people from different backgrounds and in diverse contexts draw upon different resources to live a good life.
- Salutogenic questions can help to understand how additional aspects of young people's uses of social media can be regarded as good for their health, but also how other aspects can be barriers for health development.
- There are health risks connected to social media and young people, but not necessarily the risks parents/guardians, teachers, and other adults identify as the risks.
- There is a pedagogical potential for education on, about, and through social media regarding health in a wider sense in terms of letting young people explore how social media can be a part of living a good life.
- Critical inquiry, public pedagogy and a focus on educative aspects of social media can be a way to discuss the development of a salutogenic digital citizenship education.

References

Andersson, E. and Öhman, J., 2017. Young people's conversations about environmental and sustainability issues in social media. *Environmental Education Research*, 23, 465–485.

Antonovsky, A., 1979. *Health, Stress and Coping*. San Francisco: Jossey-Bass.

Antonovsky, A., 1987. *Unravelling the Mystery of Health*. San Francisco: Jossey-Bass.

Antonovsky, A., 1996. The salutogenic model as a theory to guide health promotion. *Health Promotion International*, 32(1), 11–18.

Ericson, H., Quennerstedt, M., Skoog, T., and Johansson, M., 2017. Health resources, ageing and physical activity: A study of physically active women aged 69–75 years. *Qualitative Research in Sport, Exercise and Health*, 10(2), 206–222.

Eriksson, M., 2007. *Unravelling the Mystery of Salutogenesis: The Evidence Base of the Salutogenic Research as Measured by Antonovsky's Sense of Coherence Scale*. PhD thesis.

Evans, J., Davies, B., and Wright, J., 2004. *Body Knowledge and Control: Studies in the Sociology of Physical Education and Health*. London: Routledge.

Fitzpatrick, K. and Tinning, R., 2014. Health education's fascist tendencies: A cautionary exposition. *Critical Public Health*, 24(2), 132–142.

Gard, M. and Wright, J. 2001. Managing uncertainty: Obesity discourses and physical education in a risk society. *Studies in Philosophy and Education*, 20(6) 535–549.

Gard, M. and Wright, J., 2005. *The Obesity Epidemic: Science, Morality and Ideology*. New York: Routledge.Giroux, H.A., 2003. Public pedagogy and the politics of resistance: Notes on a critical theory of educational struggle. *Educational Philosophy and Theory*, 35(1), 5–16.

Harris, J., Cale, L., Duncombe, R., and Musson, H., 2016. Young people's knowledge and understanding of health, fitness and physical activity: Issues, divides and dilemmas. *Sport, Education and Society*, 17(2), 143–151.

Lawy, R. and Biesta, G., 2006. Citizenship-as-practice: The educational implications of an inclusive and relational understanding of citizenship. *British Journal of Educational Studies*, 54(1), 34–50.

Leahy, D., O'Flynn, G., and Wright, J., 2013. A critical 'critical inquiry' proposition in health and physical education. *Asia-Pacific Journal of Health, Sport and Physical Education*, 4(2), 175–187.

Lindström, B. and Eriksson, M., 2010. *The Hitchhiker's Guide to Salutogenesis: Salutogenic Pathways to Health Promotion*. Helsinki: Folkhälsan Research Center, Health Promotion Research.

Lupton, D., 2012. *Medicine as Culture: Illness, Disease and the Body*. London: Sage.

Macdonald, D., 2013. The new Australian health and physical education curriculum: A case of/for gradualism in curriculum reform? *Asia-Pacific Journal of Health, Sport and Physical Education*, 4(2), 95–108.

McCuaig, L. and Quennerstedt, M., 2018. Health by stealth – exploring the sociocultural dimensions of salutogenesis for sport, health and physical education research. *Sport, Education and Society*, 23(2), 111–122.

McCuaig, L., Quennerstedt, M., and Macdonald, D., 2013. A salutogenic, strengths-based approach as a theory to guide HPE curriculum change. *Asia-Pacific Journal of Health, Sport and Physical Education*, 4(2), 109–125.

Mittelmark, M.B., Sagy, S., Eriksson, M., Bauer, G.F., Pelikan, J.M., Lindström, B., and Espnes, G.A., 2017. *The Handbook of Salutogenesis*. New York: Springer.

Mossberger, K., Tolbert, C.J., and McNeal, R.S., 2007. *Digital Citizenship: The Internet, Society, and Participation*. Cambridge, MA: MIT Press.

Mossberger, K., 2009. Toward digital citizenship. Addressing inequality in the information age. *In:* A. Chadwick, ed., *Routledge Handbook of Internet Politics*. London: Routledge, 173–185.

Nordenfeldt, L., 1987. On the nature of health: An action theoretic approach. *In:* T. Beauchampt and L. Walters, eds., *Contemporary Issues in Bioethics*. Belmont CA: Wadsworth Publishing, 54–59.

Petherick, L., 2015. Shaping the child as a healthy child: Health surveillance, schools, and biopedagogies. *Cultural Studies? Critical Methodologies*, 15(5), 361–370.

Powell, D. and Fitzpatrick, K., 2015. 'Getting fit basically just means, like, nonfat': Children's lessons in fitness and fatness. *Sport, Education and Society*, 20(4), 463–484.

Przybylski, A.K., Murayama, K., DeHaan, C.R., and Gladwell, V., 2013. Motivational, emotional, and behavioral correlates of fear of missing out. *Computers in Human Behavior*, 29(4), 1841–1848.

Queensland Curriculum & Assessment Authority (2017) Health 2019 v1.1 General Senior Syllabus. Available at: www.qcaa.qld.edu.au/downloads/portal/syllabuses/snr_health_19_syll.pdf (accessed 7 December 2017).

Quennerstedt, M., 2010. Warning: physical education can seriously harm your health: But it all depends on your health perspective!. *In:* S. Brown, ed., *Issues and Controversies in Physical Education: Policy, Power and Pedagogy*. Auckland: Pearson Education, 46–56.

Quennerstedt, M., 2008. Exploring the relation between physical activity and health – a salutogenic approach to physical education. *Sport, Education and Society*, 13(3), 267–283.

Quennerstedt, M., Burrows, L., and Maivorsdotter, N., 2010. From teaching young people to be healthy to learning health. *Utbildning och Demokrati*, 19(2), 97–112.

Rydström, J., 2003. *Sinners and Citizens: Bestiality and Homosexuality in Sweden, 1880–1950*. Chicago: University of Chicago Press.

Tengland, P., 2007. Empowerment: A goal or a means for health promotion. *Medicine, Health Care and Philosophy*, 10, 197.

Tones, K. and Green, J., 2004. *Health Promotion: Planning and Strategies*. London: Sage.

WHO (1986) *The Ottawa Charter for Health Promotion*. Available at: www.who.int (accessed 17 April 2008).

Wright, J. and Burrows, L., 2004. 'Being healthy': The discursive construction of health in New Zealand children's responses to the National Education Monitoring Project. *Discourse: Studies in the Cultural Politics of Education*, 25(2), 211–230.

9 School physical education and learning about health

Pedagogical strategies for using social media

David Kirk

Chapter overview

This chapter considers school physical education, pedagogical strategies, and the role of social media in supporting young people's learning about health. I consider what can be learned from the case studies (Chapters 2–7), the wider research literature, and some of the implications for pedagogical strategies and teachers' professional learning. I conclude that physical educators can contribute to young people's critical health literacy, develop pedagogies of affect, and deploy social media forms and contents in critical and positive ways. This work will be challenging in the face of the pervasive influence of social media in young people's lives.

School physical education

School physical education has been well-established in the core curricula of many school systems since the middle of the twentieth century, and is widely recognised to provide young people with opportunities to develop their knowledge and skills in the main aspects of the physical culture of society, including sport, dance, and active leisure activities (Kirk 2010). While learning in, about, and through movement is the signal feature of most physical education programmes around the world (Arnold 1979), it is also recognised that physical education offers opportunities for education about, and the promotion of, young people's health (Quennerstedt 2008). There have been rising concerns about the emergence of social media as an increasingly prominent source of health-related information for young people, and suggestions that such uses of social media can have a negative impact on mental health (Goodyear *et al.* 2018). In this context, physical educators are being challenged to consider how they might be more reliable and authoritative sources of health-related information for young people, and so better facilitate their mental health and wellbeing (McCuaig and Quennerstedt 2016). Despite holistic definitions of physical education encompassing physical, social, cognitive, and affective dimensions of learning (Bailey *et al.* 2009), in reality physical educators have tended to focus on the physical benefits of exercise (McKenzie and Lounsbery 2009). They have also tended to see affective, social, and cognitive outcomes as by-products of participation in physical activities. As I will argue here, with only a few exceptions, physical educators have lacked examples of pedagogical approaches aiming specifically to address affective issues, such as motivation, resilience, and positive body image.

In countries like the UK, a significant amount of public funding supports secondary school programmes of physical education, with specialist teachers and facilities in most schools (Hardman 2005). Public concerns about the emotional and mental health and wellbeing of young people have prompted governments to seek new pathways to facilitate health and wellbeing (e.g. House of Commons 2017). Physical education represents one site that may be underused for this purpose, with programmes in their current form unfit for purpose (Haerens *et al.* 2011). New thinking is required around the pedagogies needed to facilitate health and wellbeing in school physical education settings, including how to teach young people about social media as an increasingly prominent source of health-related information with both positive and negative aspects.

The purpose of this chapter is to consider some pedagogical strategies that physical education teachers might develop and implement to address concerns about the role of social media in young people's health. In the first part of the chapter, I consider what we can learn about young people, social media, and health from the case studies developed from Goodyear *et al.*'s (2018) research and the wider research literature. In the second part of the chapter, I explore some of the implications of what we have learned from this literature for the development of new pedagogical strategies, and for physical education teachers' professional learning needs to implement these strategies. A key conclusion is that physical educators can play a role in developing young people's critical health literacy through pedagogies that take the affective domain as their central and explicit concern, and through teaching about the ways in which social media forms influence their physical education content. Only some of this work is currently underway and it represents a considerable challenge for physical educators in the face of the pervasive influence of social media in young people's everyday lives.

Physical education, young people, social media, and health

In this section, I consider two key points illustrated by the case studies: (i) the positioning of 'young people' as a homogenous social category and (ii) the nature of the form and content of media.

Case study analysis

This chapter, as with the others in this book, takes as a starting point the six case studies (Chapters 2–7) of young people's engagements with social media and a range of health-related issues.

Much writing in physical education and health and wellbeing conveys an impression that 'young people' can be viewed as a uniform, homogenous category that would suit a one-size-fits-all approach to research and pedagogy.

For example, Gard (2004) has been a particularly vociferous critic of the obesity lobby's insistence that 'everyone everywhere' is at risk of becoming obese. He is right to be critical because this is not so. Children living in multiple-deprivation have a considerably greater risk of becoming obese than their less deprived counterparts (Bromley *et al.* 2017). Like obesity, neither is the risk of harm from social media use uniform. Certainly, young people from all parts of society experience similar hazards in everyday life, but not equally. Indeed, the methodology of constructing the case studies to create 'individuals' who typify particular and diverse ways of engaging with social media makes this point clearly. The key message is that young people use and experience social media differently.

When we use the term 'young people', then, we do so with the understanding that the individuals and groups we are referring to experience social media in similar ways, but that the effects of this use will be mediated differently between groups and individuals by family, friends and peer group, school, neighbour-hood, local cultures, and levels of deprivation. As the case studies taken together show, social media use is complex and, as such, there will be no simple pedago-gical solutions to minimising harm and optimising good for the purposes of edu-cating about health and wellbeing.

A second point is that the nature of social media, its form and content, com-pounds this complexity. Postman (1985) reveals the issue of the form and content of media elegantly. Although he was writing as an expert on communi-cation and technology in an analogue age, Postman was at root concerned with a fundamental shift in public communication from words to images, from the Age of Typography to the Age of Television. He was concerned, moreover, by what he saw as the trivialising effect of this shift on culture and society. He argued that the way something gets communicated affects *what* gets communicated. Referring to Marshall McLuhan's famous aphorism 'the medium is the message' (Postman 1985, p. 8), Postman proposed that if this is so, it would be relatively straightforward to decipher these messages. Experience suggests otherwise, and Postman (1985, p. 10) claims instead that 'the medium is the metaphor'. Media do not simply deliver messages; meaning is often opaque, and has to be inter-preted. Nor is social media as a highly visual form of communication a source of influence by itself. Its content reflects many aspects of daily life, which the form of the medium reconfigures, distorts, or amplifies.

Two examples might suffice to demonstrate Postman's insight that form effects content. The first is from Postman's 1985 book *Amusing Ourselves to Death*. He suggests that whatever use American Indians had for smoke signals, it was highly unlikely to be for philosophical analysis. As he wrote:

> Puffs of smoke are insufficiently complex to express ideas on the nature of existence, and even if they were, a Cherokee philosopher would run short of wood or blankets long before he reached his second axiom. You cannot use smoke to do philosophy. Its form excludes the content.
>
> (Postman, 1985, p. 7)

To provide another example a little closer to our topic, we might refer to the WhatsApp conversation among the young people based on this project's data in Chapter 7. On the face of it, it is a good idea to put young people's voices into a social media form such as a WhatsApp conversation. At the same time, there is a tension around the authenticity of the conversation. The young people may indeed use this kind of social media to complain about school assemblies, teachers, and parents who don't understand the challenges they face, and some of their words may well be 'real' rather than 'fake', that is, from the data rather than the researcher's imagination. But the medium provided by WhatsApp doesn't easily facilitate this kind of 'serious' conversation. There seem to be more words than would typically make up a WhatsApp chat between a group of friends, and fewer images and emojis. It is all too reflective and reverent for a medium that encourages spontaneity and irreverent humour. At the very least, the form of the conversation risks subverting its authenticity and its persuasiveness.

The case studies (Chapters 2–7) further exemplify these two points about heterogeneity of young people and the form and content of a medium. Comparing ourselves to our peers is something people have always done and doesn't happen solely through social media. However, this activity takes on a specific shape in social media, encouraging Jess (Chapter 6), for example, to Photoshop selfies in order to look like the 'fake celebs' she admires. Wanting to be liked by others is also a commonplace human sentiment. Yet, James' (Chapter 5) use of social media takes this commonplace into a new realm; of competition between him and his peers to have the most 'likes'. And we can see here even in the notion of 'likes' an example of Postman's argument that the shift from words to images and the media that support this shift can lead to a trivialisation of content. Thus, the natural desire for peer endorsement becomes a competition for 'likes'. James' (Chapter 5) case also shows how this distortion of a commonplace human sentiment can cause inadvertent harm to someone James 'liked' only to discover he was part of 'skinny shaming' a girl who had lost weight.

For Kelly (Chapter 2), social media facilitates peer interaction and maintaining relationships. Social media keeps her 'connected'. Because of how social media works, however, by using algorithms to customise images and sites accessed by her friends, she is regularly receiving messages and images she herself didn't look for. The commentary on this and some of the other case studies expresses concern about 'the invasion of young people's social media networks by commercial parties'. The concern here, rightly, is that social media facilitates the exploitation of young people. But the algorithms that are a key feature of the form of social media do more than 'sell' young people products. They also narrow choice and awareness of alternatives, as in the case of Yaz (Chapter 3) and his viewing of inappropriate muscle-building content. The posting of images by what Leah thinks of as 'skinny girls' creates peer pressure to conform to a particular body image. Then there is the question of what is real and what is fake, as Jess' (Chapter 6) case study reveals. Because of the form social media takes and the control it gives to its users over some of its features, it is possible to manufacture images and messages that are in fact false or that mislead or misinform.

In the commentaries on the case studies, both the adults and the young people identify an overarching issue, which is how to help young people discriminate between useful and harmful health-related information. How, in short, do they become critical consumers of the metaphors social media produce? Can young people in their diversity learn to decode these metaphors? Can they learn to see through fake or misleading information? Can they become aware of alternatives to the narrow range of information social media feeds them? Who is best placed to help young people, particularly when they think their teachers or parents don't understand the challenges they face? Is there a role for schools and for physical education in particular to use social media to support better health-related education for young people? The commentaries also ask whether the owners of social media sites should take greater responsibility by adopting, perhaps, a code of practice that requires them to filter inappropriate material?

Physical education literature

What do we know from the existing research literature on physical education that might help us to answer the questions posed in the previous paragraph? The short answer would appear to be 'very little'. There is little robust research evidence on how young people use social media and, in particular, how they encounter, access, and respond to information relating to health. Beyond their own research, Goodyear *et al.* (2018) note that there has been recent interest in this issue internationally (e.g. Haussmann *et al.* 2017) though there is a lack of a critical mass of robust empirical research upon which to base interventions.

A general conclusion from this work to date is that while young people are often sceptical of health-related messages and products on social media, they nevertheless lack the critical health literacy skills to make accurate judgements about the value of that information (e.g. Cusak *et al.* 2017). Researchers also report the potential for serious harm resulting from internet use generally (Marchant *et al.* 2017), from social media use in particular, and its effects on mental health (Frith 2017), from social media addiction (Webb and Wasilick 2015) and from anxieties centred on body image (Andsager 2014). Goodyear *et al.* (2018) point out the consequences of this gap in the knowledge that's available, and its availability in formats that can inform teachers, clinicians, and other health practitioners, are that there are currently limited understanding about how to design programmes that might utilise the popularity and attractions of social media for young people to positively benefit their health and wellbeing.

This information gap has not discouraged physical education researchers and teachers from positive advocacy for the use of social media in physical education. Advocates recognise the pervasiveness and power of social media and see an urgent need for physical educators to keep up with youth and 'speak their language' (e.g. Lambert 2016). At the same time, supporters of social media use in health and physical education classes do recognise the need for quality control

(Erwin 2016). Nonetheless, there is a strong positive tone to the literature as exemplified by a recent opinion forum in *JOPERD* (2017). This forum revealed that physical educators perceive wide-ranging benefits such as teachers sharing ideas, reaching out to students, promoting active lifestyles, promoting physical education in the face of budget cuts, and teachers acting as role models to students in their own use of social media. Some writers advocate the use of specific social media sites such as Pinterest (Franks and Krause 2017) and others (e.g. Polsgrove and Frimming 2013) see the creative use of social media as a means of enhancing students' health and fitness knowledge.

This enthusiasm for new tools to support learning can be regarded as admirable and it acknowledges that physical educators need to keep abreast of digital technology in general and social media in particular. There is, at the same time, little acknowledgement in this small literature of questions to be asked about teachers' suitability to make safe and appropriate use of social media as an educational tool. The idea that teachers might view themselves as role models for the use of social media is immediately problematic given what we have learned from the research underpinning the case studies in this book, particularly about young people's views of adults and their lack of understanding of the pressures young people face using social media in their everyday lives. Nevertheless, positive recognition by physical educators that social media is part of their business as educators of young people is significant since it suggests they can see the need to engage with this technology. In the next section of this chapter, I move on to explore some of the implications for physical education's contribution to educating young people about health using social media.

Implications for using social media in physical education to support young people's learning about health

In order to explore some of the implications for physical education of what has been presented so far, it is helpful to return to Postman (1985) in order to understand the scale of the challenge schools face in relation to social media form and content. To conclude his analysis in *Amusing Ourselves to Death*, Postman cites the 'Huxleyan Warning', referring to Aldous Huxley's dystopian novel *Brave New Word* (1932). He writes:

> What Huxley teaches is that in the age of advanced technology, spiritual devastation is more likely to come from an enemy with a smiling face than from one whose countenance exudes suspicion and hate. In the Huxleyan prophecy, Big Brother does not watch us, by his choice. We watch him, by ours.... When a population becomes distracted by trivia, when cultural life is re-defined as a perpetual round of entertainments, when serious public conversation becomes a form of baby-talk, when, in short, a people become an audience and their public business a vaudeville act, then a nation finds itself at risk; culture-death is a clear possibility.
>
> (Postman 1985, p. 156)

Postman was, as we noted earlier, referring to the rise of television in American society and its displacement of print as a principle form of public discourse. His overarching point was that *what* is communicated is shaped by the *form* of a medium. It takes little intellectual effort to see how Postman's analysis of a society dominated by television applies with even greater and more devastating force to one dominated by various forms of digital media, including social media. Arguably, the rise of reality TV has taken this media form to one extreme, to the extent that the current President of the United States is regularly accused of running his presidency as if he were starring in a reality TV show.[1] The fact that we learn what is on this President's mind more often through *Twitter* than any carefully crafted public statement or policy provides a measure, not just of the individual concerned, but of the extent to which such forms of digital media have penetrated society and have become normalised. Central to Postman's critique of television and, we might extrapolate, of social media, is its trivialisation of culture, and also its entertainment value.

Postman's language of 'spiritual devastation' and 'culture-death' may seem extreme, but scaled down to the level of a young person, it could be argued that it does not unreasonably overstate the nature of mental illness in the many forms associated with social media use and misuse. Marchant *et al.*'s (2017) systematic review citing earlier of internet use, self-harm, and suicidal behaviour is not the stuff of sensationalism but instead reflects the everyday realities of some young people's experiences in a digital age. Nevertheless, despite the more and less obvious manifestations of harm social media facilitates, we cannot understate its drawing power as a form of entertainment and much more. In one case study, Kelly's 'connected' narrative (Chapter 2) begins with an exclamation: 'A world without social media "are you mad?!"' As Postman cast around for solutions to the powerful and terrible conclusions he had reached, he considered then dismissed attempts by families, organisations, and state governments to limit television viewing. He sees the Luddite position (of destroying the technology) as futile. As he put it: 'Americans will not shut down any part of their technological apparatus, and to suggest that they do so is to make no suggestion at all' (Postman 1985, p. 158). We might follow the call during the Television Age to restrict viewing of certain topics (e.g. Tobacco advertising) at certain times of the day and night (e.g. The BBC's watershed for children's viewing) by requiring social media sites to work to a code of practice. This for Postman (1985, p. 160) was mere tinkering, however, since the problem was not '*what* people watch ... but *that* we watch'. The solution, he believed, was in *how* people watched television.

I am going to suggest that a similar solution applies in relation to social media use and *how* both young people and adults use it in educational contexts. In other words, we need a different order of solution to the problem than is typically called for by teachers, researchers, and young people themselves. In the next section I outline three pedagogical strategies that might be employed in physical education (often in collaboration with other fields) in relation to using social media to support education about health in physical education.

Pedagogical strategies in physical education

One pedagogical strategy already widely advocated in the literature is to facilitate the development of young people's health literacy (Nutbeam 2008). Interactive and critical health literacy, that is, the ability to extract key information from various sources and to subject it to critical scrutiny, would appear to offer an important starting point for the work schools might do. Physical education teachers have a clear part to play here since there is a pressing need for the accuracy of health-related information and the trustworthiness of sources.

There are two issues to consider with this strategy. One is that physical education programmes in their current form do not necessarily provide the propositional knowledge and associated analytical skills underpinning the development of critical health literacy (Kirk 2010). Indeed, where they do provide this information, it is usually in relation to the training effects of exercise on the body which they deliver informally and incidentally, integrated into practical physical activity units. Typically, physical education teachers don't address sensitive issues such as body image (Kerner *et al.* 2017), but these appear to be regularly occurring concerns for young people in social media contexts.

A second issue relates to heterogeneity among young people. Indeed, Leah's (Chapter 4) and Yaz's (Chapter 3) different health-related information needs and interests illustrate this in relation to the same topic, body image. The challenge for teachers adopting this first pedagogical strategy – health literacy – is to provide the information underpinning health literacy in ways that meet the needs of individuals and groups of individuals. This in turn requires a different approach to the teacher-led pedagogies that are regular features of most physical education classes (Kirk 2010), a matter addressed in the second strategy.

In order to get to the second strategy, it is worth reminding ourselves that the issues with social media use and young people, as illustrated by the case studies, most often relate to mental health and wellbeing. This is what physical educators would typically refer to as the 'affective domain', populated with matters of motivation, resilience, perceived physical competence, body image, enjoyment, interest, and coping (Metzler 2017). A second strategy, then, is to develop what might be called 'pedagogies of affect', pedagogical strategies that take the affective domain as their explicit and central concern. The bad news is that, with only a few examples, physical educators have a poor track-record in this domain. While the affective domain has been recognised as part of the business of physical education, traditionally, learning has been viewed as a by-product of programmes rather than a central and explicit objective. Enjoyment, resilience, motivation, perseverance, and the rest are hoped, rather than planned, for.

We can count among the few well-established examples of pedagogies of affect in physical education: Siedentop's (1994) Sport Education model, Hellison's (2003) Teaching Personal and Social Responsibility approach (TPSR) and Oliver's Activist Approach to working with adolescent girls (Oliver and Kirk 2015). Some may wish to argue for inclusion of Cooperative Learning (e.g. Dyson and Casey 2016) on this list, and while it is certainly a pedagogy of affect and used in physical education programmes, arguably it is not a model specific to physical education.

The Activist Approach, built on over 20 years of Kim Oliver's pathfinding work, provides an illustrative example of what a pedagogy of affect looks like in physical education, and contrasts markedly with traditional physical education practice. A critical element of the Activist pedagogical model is student-centeredness whereby listening to girls' voices is crucial, as is responding to them constructively. During a recently completed pilot project based in four Glasgow schools (Kirk *et al.* 2018), we sought, in Cook-Sather's (2002) terms, to 'authorise student voice', which involved a shift in the power dynamic between teachers and pupils. Another feature of this Activist Approach is pedagogies of embodiment. Here, teachers worked with girls to co-create an environment where girls felt comfortable to engage whole-heartedly in physical education activities, where they could trust their teacher and other girls not to judge them. Perseverance was encouraged by this enhanced level of engagement. Pedagogies of embodiment featured prominently in the project data since the moving body is the central object of physical education (Standal 2015). Comfort and confidence, trust and not feeling judged were, for the girls in the study, key to their physical education experience.

Pedagogies of affect do not address social media use directly, but they create environments in physical education classes that make it possible for the kinds of issues that social media amplifies and distorts, such as relationships, perceptions of the body, perceived physical competence, power dynamics, and so on, to be addressed explicitly and sensitively. They also recognise the importance of how young people feel about themselves and others, how they treat themselves and others, and the nature of their embodiment, particularly in visible and public settings such as school physical education.

Physical educators might also take forward a third pedagogical strategy in relation to social media, young people, and health. Here, though, they will undoubtedly need to collaborate with teachers who have expertise in the ways in which social media works because this strategy would involve critical literacy skills not just in relation to the content of social media, but to the form of the medium itself. Postman (1985, p. 161) argued that: 'No medium is excessively dangerous if its users understand what its dangers are'. His point is that it is in itself empowering to understand how the form of a medium shapes a message. What is required in this strategy, then, is educating young people about the relationships between social media forms and content. Given physical education teachers' knowledge of (some) health-related content, they would be essential collaborators in providing such programmes.

The case studies reported by Goodyear *et al.* (2018) provide many examples of how form shapes content in social media. The ways in which algorithms select the information that appears on social media sites, often unlooked for by individual members of groups, are referred to in two cases. In Kelly's case (Chapter 2), they operate through the Search and Explore function,[2] and leave her vulnerable to exploitation by commercial interests, while in Yaz's case

(Chapter 3) the algorithms work increasingly to narrow the information he receives. Both Yaz's (Chapter 3) and Leah's cases (Chapter 4) reveal how the visual dominates the social media sites they use. James' (Chapter 5) competition to accumulate as many 'likes' as possible and the way in which this contributed to harming someone else exemplifies how social media trivialises the whole idea of friendship, or being liked for who you are. What is 'real' and what is 'fake' become genuine dilemmas for young people such as Jess (Chapter 6), contributing to the normalisation of a 'post-truth' era (Klein 2017), while at the same time rendering problematic the trustworthiness of information and the notion of 'expertise'. Kelly's (Chapter 2) case reveals the up and down sides of instantaneous connectedness, while Yaz (Chapter 3) is able to claim he prefers information from social media because it is simplified and there are no 'information essays'.

This selection of examples from the case studies show that it is possible to analyse and critique the *form* that is social media and its effects on content. But for schools to open up conversations with young people around this topic may be fraught with difficulties. Not only does the task require collaboration among teachers across the school, it requires adults to be credible and knowledgeable about young people's experiences of social media, and not just its health-related content. Critique may be painful for young people if it requires them to give up the pleasures social media provide. Moreover, as Postman (1985, p. 162) again noted: 'To ask of our schools that they engage in the task of de-mythologizing media is to ask something the schools have never done'. His reference here is to the critique and de-mythologizing of print media in terms of how form and content interact. His point provides a glimpse of the scale of the challenge for the development of critical health literacy in schools centred on digital media.

Professional learning needs for teachers

It is commonplace in the current educational climate to regard initial teacher education as a starting point in a teacher's professional development, with an expectation in many education systems that professional learning will be a career-long process (Korthagen 2005). This is an important development now that in many education systems the initial professional preparation of physical education teachers is limited to a one- to two-year postgraduate programme, with much of this school-based. A consensus also seems to have emerged that by far the most effective form of teacher professional learning is in the workplace itself, supported by peers and by other stakeholders in teacher education such as universities, local education authorities and school inspectors (MacPhail *et al.* 2014). Career-long teacher professional learning is then the context in which we should consider how we provide for teachers to learn new pedagogical strategies for young people, social media, and health. All three of the strategies outlined in the previous section have implications for teacher professional learning.

With respect to facilitating interactive and critical health literacy, most physical education teachers will by virtue of having completed undergraduate degrees in sport and exercise sciences or a related topic be able to provide a sound and trustworthy source of health-related information on the effects of exercise on the body, both for sport performance and health and wellbeing. Some of their undergraduate preparation may include psychological as well as biophysical knowledge and, perhaps less often, sociocultural understanding of health and wellbeing. While this is a valuable resource physical educators can bring to this first strategy, as we noted, some consideration would be required of how teachers could provide this resource in the face of traditional practice, particularly where it is carried out informally and incidentally within practical physical activity units.

Teachers' professional learning needs here will focus on how to plan for the provision of the propositional knowledge and analytical skills underpinning interactive and critical health literacy, at the same time acknowledging students' differentiated needs and interests. Workplace-based professional learning is important with respect to differentiation since the local context in which health literacy is to be applied informs teacher learning. Physical education teachers may need support, however, to learn to deal with topics with which hitherto they have had little experience, such as body image.

Pedagogies of affect present an altogether bigger challenge for physical educators in terms of their professional learning. As we already noted, there are few well-established examples of approaches to physical education that make affective learning aspirations explicit and central, and neither are the approaches that exist widely practiced. The teachers in the Activist pilot project in Glasgow did learn over the course of a year to practice pedagogies of affect that had clear educational benefits for the adolescent girls they worked with (Kirk *et al.* 2018). We reported that it was only through the experience of working with an Activist Approach in their schools over time that the teachers learned what worked and what didn't, learned about their pupils, learned from other teachers, and learned about themselves. We also found that the teachers developed relationships with their pupils and the girls with each other that were stronger and more trusting than they had been able to formerly. This is important if teachers and pupils are to co-create a learning environment that allows confidence, enjoyment, and motivation but also the concerns and fears that require perseverance and resilience to be acknowledged openly and resolved collectively.

The third strategy, of teaching about how the form of social media affects its contents, would appear at first glance to fall outside the remit of physical education teachers. Perhaps teachers in fields such as ICT are better placed to lead on this strategy. Nevertheless, since young people are encountering health-related information through social media and physical education teachers represent a source of expertise on this topic, we might argue that they should at least be partners in this strategy. In order to do this, we might argue further that all teachers should at least be familiar with social media forms. This doesn't mean that teachers should become users themselves of social media, but they will need a level of first-hand experience to understand how this technology works and is used by young people, and for the development of their professional critical literacy skills. This professional learning need is not just to contribute to teaching social media literacy, but also to being credible with their pupils.

Postman (1985) commented that schools have never engaged in this task, at least in a systematic way that takes seriously the influence on the form of a medium of communication, not just on the content and meaning of the messages it conveys, but on the ways in which users of that medium think. This is not a technical task, then, of critiquing media, to be left to media specialists. It may be that ICT teachers would find it difficult to gain the analytic distance from their area of expertise to be critical of its forms. There are, consequently, wider issues here for teacher professional learning across the whole curriculum since social media's influence is everywhere.

This means that physical education teachers must be part of a pedagogical strategy that seeks to teach about social media's form and content. The enthusiasm of the contributors to the *JOPERD* forum for physical educators to engage with social media is admirable, but this cannot be done uncritically. Quality control, as Erwin (2016) outlined, will undoubtedly be important in physical educators' embrace of social media. It is crucial for teacher professional learning that the reasons for doing so are clear. 'Speaking their language', as Lambert (2016) urges, may be important for teachers' credibility with young people. But learning to do so must also be for teachers to better understand social media form and content in order to de-mythologize it, a far more challenging task. Part of their professional learning will also have to be how to support young people in their diversity when their sources of entertainment, connection, and information are the object of critical analysis.

Summary of key messages

- Young people experience social media in similar ways, but unequally. There is evidence to show, in the case studies and elsewhere in the research literature, that social media can be both harmful and beneficial to young people's health and wellbeing. The effects of social media on health are mediated differently between groups and individuals by family, friends and peer group, school, neighbourhood, local cultures, and levels of deprivation.
- The form social media take influences content, in ways that reconfigure, trivialise, distort, or amplify messages about a wide range of matters that impact on health and wellbeing.
- The research literature can provide some insights into young people's uses of social media but much more needs to be known before we can develop effective interventions that help minimise harm and optimise benefits to young people's health and wellbeing.
- Three pedagogical strategies are proposed that physical educators and teachers in other curricular areas could implement to assist young people with social media, the development of health literacy, the development of

pedagogies of affect, and teaching explicitly and critically about the ways in which the social media forms influence content.

• Teachers of physical education will have professional learning needs in order to develop and implement these pedagogical strategies.

Notes

1 www.nationalreview.com/g-file/448716/donald-trumps-reality-tv-presidency-cross overs
2 We're always working to update the types of photos and videos you see in Search & Explore to better tailor it to you. Posts are selected automatically based on things like the people you follow or the posts you like. You may also see video channels, which can include posts from a mixture of hand-picked and automatically sourced accounts based on topics we think you'll enjoy (https://help.instagram. com/487224561296752)

References

Andsager, J.L., 2014. Research directions in social media and body image. *Sex Roles*, 71, 407–413.
Arnold, P.J., 1979. *Meaning in Movement, Sport and Physical Education*. London: Heinemann.
Bailey, R., Armour, K., Kirk, D., Jess, M., Pickup, I., and Sandford, R., 2009. The educational benefits claimed for physical education and school sport: An academic review. *Research Papers in Education*, 24(1), 1–27.
Bromley, C., Tod, E., and McCartney, G., 2017. *Obesity and Health Inequalities in Scotland: Summary Report*. Edinburgh: NHS Health Scotland.
Cook-Sather, A., 2002. Authorizing students' perspectives: Toward trust, dialogue, and change in education. *Educational Researcher*, 3(4), 3–14.
Cusak, L., Desha, L.N., Del Mar, C.B., and Hoffman, T.C., 2017. A qualitative study exploring high school students' understanding of, and attitudes towards, health information and claims. *Health Expectations*, 20, 1163–1171.
Dyson, B. and Casey, A., 2016. *Cooperative Learning in Physical Education and Physical Activity: A Practical Introduction*. London: Routledge.
Erwin, H., 2016. The use of social media by physical educators: How do we ensure quality control? *Journal of Physical Education, Recreation & Dance*, 87, 2.
Franks, H. and Krause, J.M., 2017. Winning with pinning: Enhancing health and physical education with Pinterest. *Journal of Physical Education, Recreation & Dance*, 88(5), 15–19.
Frith, E., 2017. Social media and children's mental health: A review of the evidence. Accessed from: https://epi.org.uk/wp-content/uploads/2017/06/Social-Media_Mental-Health_EPI-Report.pdf
Gard, M., 2004. An elephant in the room and a bridge too far, or physical education and the 'obesity epidemic'. *In:* J. Evans, B. Davies, and J. Wright, eds., *Body Knowledge and Control: Studies in the Sociology of Physical Education and Health*. London: Routledge, 68–82.
Goodyear, V., Armour, K., and Wood, H., 2018. Young people and their engagement with health-related social media: New perspectives. *Sport, Education and Society*, iFirst Article.

Haerens, L., Kirk, D., Cardon, G., and Bourdeauhuji, I., 2011. The development of a pedagogical model for Health-Based Physical Education. *Quest*, 63, 321–338.

Hardman, K. 2005. *Foreword. In:* E. Puhse and M. Gerber, eds., *International Comparison of Physical Education: Concepts, Problems, Prospects.* Oxford: Meyer, 12–17.

Haussmann, J.D., Touloumtzis, C., White, M.T., Colbert, M.D., and Golding, H.C., 2017. Adolescent and young adult use of social media for health and its implications. *Journal of Adolescent Health*, 60(6), 714–719.

Hellison, D., 2003. *Teaching Responsibility through Physical Activity.* Champaign, IL.: Human Kinetics.

House of Commons Education and Health Committees. 2017. *Children and Young People's Mental Health – the Role of Education.* London: House of Commons.

JOPERD. 2017. Is social media (Twitter, Facebook, etc.) a positive thing for physical education/health teachers to engage in? Why or why not?, *Journal of Physical Education, Recreation & Dance*, 88(6), 63–67.

Kerner, C., Haerens, L., and Kirk, D., 2017. Understanding body image in physical education: current knowledge and future directions, *European Physical Education Review*, Published Online ahead of print, DOI: 10.1177/1356336X17692508

Kirk, D., 2010. *Physical Education Futures.* London: Routledge.

Kirk, D., Lamb, C.A., Oliver, K.L. with Ewing-Day, R., Fleming, C., Loch, A., and Smedley, V., 2018. Balancing prescription and teacher and pupil agency: Spaces for manoeuvre within a pedagogical model for working with adolescent girls. *The Curriculum Journal*, iFirst Article.

Klein, N., 2017. *No is Not Enough: Defeating the New Shock Politics.* London: Allen Lane.

Korthagen, F., 2005. Practice, theory and person in life-long professional leaning. *In:* D. Beijaard, P.C., Merjer, G. Morine-Dershimer, and T. Harm, eds., *Teacher Professional Development in Changing Conditions.* New York: Springer, 79–94.

Lambert, C., 2016. Technology has a place in physical education, *Journal of Physical Education, Recreation & Dance*, 87, 9.

MacPhail, A., Patton, K., Parker, M., and Tannehill, D., 2014. Leading by EXAMPLE: Teacher educators' professional learning through Communities of Practice. *Quest*, 66, 39–56.

Marchant, A., Hawton, K., Stewart, A., Montgomery, P., Singaravelu, V., Lloyd, K., Purdy, N., Daine, K., and John, A., 2017. A systematic review of the relationship between internet use, self-harm and suicidal behaviour in young people: The good, the bad and the unknown. *PLoS ONE* 12(8), e0181722.

McCuaig, L. and Quennerstedt, M., 2016. Health by stealth – exploring the sociocultural dimensions of salutogenesis for sport, health and physical education research. *Sport, Education and Society*, 23(2), 111–122.

McKenzie, T.L. and Lounsbery, M.A., 2009. School physical education: The pill not taken. *American Journal of Lifestyle Education*, 3, 219–225.

Metzler, M.W., 2017. *Instructional Models for Physical Education.* London: Routledge.

Nutbeam, D., 2008. The evolving concept of health literacy. *Social Science and Medicine*, 67, 2072–2078.

Oliver, K.L. and Kirk, D., 2015. *Girls, Gender and Physical Education: An Activist Approach.* London: Routledge.

Polsgrove, M.J. and Frimming, R.E., 2013/ A creative way to utilize social media to enhance fitness and health knowledge. *Strategies*, 26, 3–7.

Postman, N., 1985. *Amusing Ourselves to Death: Public discourse in the Age of Show Business*. Harmondsworth: Penguin.

Quennerstedt, M., 2008. Exploring the relation between physical activity and health – a salutogenic approach to physical education. *Sport, Education and Society*, 13(3), 267–283.

Siedentop, D., 1994. *Sport Education: Quality PE through Positive Sport Experiences*. Champaign, IL.: Human Kinetics.

Standal, O.F., 2015. *Phenomenology and Pedagogy in Physical Education*. London: Routledge.

Webb, M.C. and Wasilick, L.M., 2015. Addressing social media addiction via the classroom. *Journal of Health Education Teaching Techniques*, 2 (3), 1–9.

10 Young people, social media, and disordered eating

Anthony Papathomas, Hannah J. White, and Carolyn R. Plateau

Chapter overview

In this chapter we explore whether adolescent social media practices can contribute to disordered eating attitudes and behaviours. Drawing on the case study data (Chapters 2–7), we connect adolescents' accounts of their social media experiences to the disordered eating risk-factor literature. Our analysis proposes three principal themes for consideration: (1) Social media-induced body dissatisfaction; (2) Self(ie)-objectification practices; and (3) Health and nutrition Insta-norms. These themes illuminate specific processes by which young people might develop dangerous eating patterns as a result of interacting online. To conclude, we offer a series of practical strategies to temper social media-induced disordered eating risks.

Disordered eating

Disordered eating encompasses a continuum of problematic eating attitudes and behaviours spanning unhealthy dieting through to clinically diagnosed eating disorders (Shisslak, Crago, and Estes 1995). Anorexia nervosa (AN) and bulimia nervosa (BN) represent severe and difficult to treat illnesses that lie at the extreme end of this continuum. The fifth edition of the Diagnostic and Statistical Manual of Mental Disorders (DSM-V, American Psychiatric Association 2013) details the core clinical features associated with AN and BN. For AN, self-starvation leads to body weight that is less than minimally expected for a person's age and height. BN is characterised by binge-eating episodes whereby a large amount of food is consumed while experiencing a loss of control. To prevent weight gain, the individual then 'purges' via self-induced vomiting or through the use of laxatives. The DSM-V highlights that both AN and BN are underpinned by irrational beliefs, such as an intense fear of gaining weight, excessive influence of body shape or weight on self-evaluation, and disturbed perceptions of their bodies. Although AN and BN dominate public consciousness, a wide range of subclinical disordered eating conditions exist and these also present physical and mental distress (Wade *et al.* 2012). Further, subclinical disordered eating is much more pervasive than AN or BN (see subsequent section) and it therefore represents a public health issue in its own right.

Eating disorder onset and prevalence

Adolescence has been outlined as the critical period for the development of eating disorders (Striegel-Moore and Bulik 2007). The highest reported rates of both AN and BN are among ten to 19 year olds (Currin *et al.* 2005). Specifically, 5.7 per cent of adolescent girls report an eating disorder diagnosis in their lifetime compared with 1.2 per cent of adolescent boys (Smink *et al.* 2014). Prevalence estimates are typically conceived as 'underestimates' however due to the limits of self-report and the stigma associated with disclosing mental illness (Papathomas and Lavallee 2012). This is particularly the case for males due to the embarrassment caused by cultural conceptions of eating disorders as a female disease (see Papathomas 2014). Further, the true extent of the problem comes to light when prevalence captures subclinical issues that lie further down the disordered eating continuum. For example, in a study that asked adolescents to report behaviour over the previous 12 months, 49.3 per cent of girls and 37.8 per cent of boys had engaged in unhealthy weight control behaviours, such as skipping meals or fasting (Eisenberg *et al.* 2012).

Disordered eating risk factors

The dominant focus of research into disordered eating has been on risk factors (Papathomas and Lavallee 2012). Risk-factor research seeks to identify social, psychological, or biological factors implicated in the cause of disordered eating (Striegel-Moore and Bulik 2007). We now go on to discuss some of the major disordered eating risk factors identified in the literature.

Body dissatisfaction

Body dissatisfaction typically occurs when there is a perceived discrepancy between a person's actual body and their ideal body; the larger the discrepancy, the greater the body dissatisfaction (Grogan 2016). In adolescence, body dissatisfaction can predict dieting and disordered weight control behaviours five years later (Neumark-Sztainer *et al.* 2006). Further, adolescents who feel bad about their bodies also demonstrate more low self-esteem and depressive symptoms (Paxton *et al.* 2006). For some, body dissatisfaction is the most salient factor in the development of disordered eating practices (Stice, Marti, and Durant 2011). Certain factors can lead to increased body dissatisfaction, such as perceived pressure to be thin and the internalisation of unrealistic thin ideals (Stice and Whitenton 2002).

Internalisation of the thin ideal

Within Western cultures, both men and women are subject to a narrow, socially constructed view of what is considered physically attractive. For females, the feminine thin ideal portrays slenderness as the ultimate indicator of beauty

(Swami 2015). The masculine ideal dictates that attractiveness is characterised by the presence of large and well-defined musculature in combination with low body fat and a narrow waist (Griffiths, Murray, and Touyz 2013). These pervasive body norms work to police what is considered an acceptable way to look (Erchull 2015). Through various media representations, the thin ideal also becomes synonymous with being loved, valued, and successful (Hesse-Biber *et al.* 2006). Individuals who buy in to the idea that these narrowly prescribed body types are indeed 'ideal' are said to 'internalise' them. The process of internalising a thin ideal involves integrating the cultural standard into one's belief system to the point of striving to achieve it (Thompson *et al.* 1999). It is a problematic process, however, as the thin ideal, for females at least, is below a 'normal' body weight and hence unrealistic and nearly impossible to achieve (Owen and Laurel-Seller 2000). As such, those who internalise the thin ideal often experience body dissatisfaction, stringent dieting, and low mood, which can subsequently increase the risk of disordered eating behaviours (Stice 2001). Complicating matters, there has been some movement away from a purely thin ideal to a 'thin and toned' ideal (see Benton and Karazia 2015). Although the addition of tone might be construed as positive, exposure to fit-ideal images has been associated with greater body dissatisfaction than viewing thin ideal images (Robinson *et al.* 2017).

Social pressure to be thin

Social pressures regarding weight and shape may also exist within an individual's environment. Among adolescent girls, it has been reported that parental encouragement to diet and family and peer weight teasing have been linked with dieting (Balantekin *et al.* 2018) or the use of extreme weight control behaviours, such as diet-pill or laxative use (Neumark-Sztainer *et al.* 2010). Some individuals may be more susceptible to these pressures. For example, body-dissatisfied adolescent girls reported a greater perception of influence from their friends in relation to body attitudes and weight loss behaviours (Rayner *et al.* 2013). These studies suggest that comments made by family or friends may contribute to the internalisation of thin ideals and an over-evaluation of the importance of appearance and body weight.

Self-objectification theory (see Fredrickson and Roberts 1997) argues that the objectification of female bodies by others can lead to women objectifying themselves in the same way. Essentially, when a woman is judged entirely according to her sexual attractiveness, whether positively or negatively, she may internalise this message and view her own worth as dependent on appearance to others. It is an example of how the thin ideal can be internalised through direct social interactions. Fredrickson and Robert's (1998) hypothesis was that women who view themselves as sexual objects to be admired by others will be more inclined to engage in excessive body monitoring, stringent dieting, and disordered eating. It is an assertion that continues to receive much attention and support in the literature (e.g. Adams *et al.* 2017; Cheng *et al.* 2017).

Social comparison

Social comparison theory (see Festinger 1954) outlines that individuals make social comparisons to evaluate their own opinions and abilities. This process provides feedback on a valued personal characteristic and the development of knowledge about oneself. In relation to learning more about one's appearance, meta-analytic findings suggest that greater emphasis on appearance-related social comparisons has been associated with increased body dissatisfaction (Myers and Crowther 2009). This relationship holds true when comparisons were made with peers or thin media images. Social comparisons may also influence eating behaviour, with adolescent girls more likely to be dieting if their friends are also dieting (Balentekin *et al.* 2017). Further, adolescent disordered eating and muscle-enhancing behaviour has been associated with friends' engagement in these practices (Eisenberg *et al.* 2012).

Dieting

The risk of developing an eating disorder is reported to be eight times higher among adolescent girls who diet compared with those who do not (Patton *et al.* 1999). Young people may initiate dieting due to body dissatisfaction, weight concerns, and weight importance (Mendes *et al.* 2014). Among adolescents, greater adiposity is associated with higher levels of dietary restraint and body dissatisfaction (Goldfield *et al.* 2010). Furthermore, adolescent dieting has been associated with the increased risk of engaging in extreme weight control behaviours (such as self-induced vomiting, or using laxatives or diet pills) or developing an eating disorder five years later (Neumark-Sztainer *et al.* 2006).

In summary, clinical eating disorders lie at the extreme end of a disordered eating continuum. Although less severe, subclinical disordered eating is still associated with psychological distress and it is far more prevalent than AN or BN. More females than males develop disordered eating and adolescence is the primary stage of onset. A range of risk factors predict disordered eating development and these include body dissatisfaction; internalisation of the thin ideal; social pressures to be thin, social comparisons and dieting practices. In the following section, we highlight the ways social media might contribute to the presence of such risk factors and thus the development of disordered eating.

Young people, social media, and disordered eating

Having discussed research and theory related to eating disorders, we now use this to guide our analysis of the case studies of young people's social media use (Chapters 2–7). What follows is a theoretically informed commentary of our collaborative insights into how certain forms of social media use relate to disordered eating. Each chapter author read each of the case studies independently and noted areas of conceptual interest, much like the free coding phase of many forms of qualitative data analysis (Braun *et al.* 2016). We then met as a group to discuss and challenge respective interpretations and, where relevant, co-construct new ones. This process was not deployed as a strategy to claim our reading is 'correct' or the 'only plausible reading', but to ensure our interpretive efforts were rigorously deliberated and stand up to interrogation (Smith and McGannon 2018).

On identifying numerous points of insight, we set about narrowing down to a number of topics suitable to be discussed in depth within the confines of the book chapter. Although this was not an easy task, given the breadth and richness of the data, the following three issues were identified as being particularly pronounced in the case studies: (i) Social media-induced body dissatisfaction, (ii) Self(ie)-objectification practices, and (iii) Health and nutrition Insta-norms. These interpretations are now discussed with reference to empirical literature and extracts from the case study chapters.

Social media-induced body dissatisfaction

Across several of the case studies, there was an overt emphasis on the capacity for social media to lead to feelings of insecurity about one's physical appearance. The case study of Leah (Chapter 4) is perhaps the most powerful demonstration of this. Leah represents a teenage female who regularly uses Instagram and who looks at images of 'skinny girls' which make her feel '10 times worse' about how her own body looks. As we have argued in the previous section, these ideals are unrealistic. According to the literature, Leah's experiences are also not unique. Viewing images of other people's bodies on social media platforms can lead to significant body dissatisfaction (e.g. Fardouly *et al.* 2015; Fardouly and Vartanian 2016; Holland and Tiggeman 2016; Tiggeman and Slater 2017). Body dissatisfaction may be particularly prevalent when social media posts portray the feminine thin ideal or the masculine muscular ideal (Carrotte, Prichard, and Lim 2017). In a systematic review of 20 studies, Holland and Tiggeman (2016) identified consistent positive relationships between social media use, body dissatisfaction, and disordered eating. Although most of the studies reviewed were simple correlations, a small number of experimental studies also showed that social media use negatively impacted body image and eating behaviour.

Of course, the notion that media portrayals of beauty can negatively influence body image and eating behaviour is not new (see Levine and Murnen 2009; López-Guimerà *et al.* 2010), but rather the *type* of media has changed. Numerous similarities exist between the ways traditional media (e.g. magazines) and contemporary media (e.g. social media) emphasise norms of attractiveness. First, idealised celebrity bodies (as seen in Chapter 6) characterise magazine and film (Botta 2003) but this has broadened to include social media sites (Brown and Tiggeman 2016). Second, both traditional and new media can be seen as conduits for *youth* fashion and culture – youth being the developmental stage where ideals about the self and how one should look begin to be internalised (Flament *et al.* 2012). Third, where professional magazines are maligned for using photo editing software to fabricate unattainable ideals (Reaves *et al.* 2004), social media users can apply 'filters' to enhance their aesthetic appeal (McLean *et al.* 2015) (see also Chapter 6). Given these similarities, efforts to understand how social media might influence disordered eating attitudes and behaviours should not be seen as totally divorced from decades of research into the role of traditional media.

In contrast, there is also much that is distinctive about social media which may intensify messages about beauty and precipitate feelings of body dissatisfaction and subsequently disordered eating. For example, social media demands more *active engagement and interaction* than either film or print media. The case studies (Chapters 2–7) illuminate the pervasiveness of social media engagement; as they report it, participants post images and updates 'all the time' about 'literally everything' and, in turn, others 'like', 'react', or 'comment' on these posts. This 'functionality' ensures social media engagement is an all-consuming experience and therefore one that can heighten homogenised portrayals of beauty beyond more passive forms of media. In support of this assertion, more time spent on Facebook is positively correlated with greater internalisation of the feminine thin ideal (Tiggeman and Slater 2013). Further, as reported by Tiggemann and Slater (2017), adolescent girls' increased uses of Facebook corresponded with increases in body image concerns. In the same study, the number of Facebook friends was also found to predict a drive for thinness. In this sense, more friends could facilitate more opportunities for negative social comparison, leading to body dissatisfaction. Because social comparisons via social media sites typically involve comparing oneself to one's peers rather than to celebrities (see Chapter 6), unfavourable verdicts may be particularly damaging to body image.

Self(ie)-objectification practices

Most of the research into social media use and disordered eating focuses on viewing unattainable bodies online and the resultant impact on wellbeing, body image, and eating behaviour (e.g. Fardouly and Vartanian 2016; Holland and Tiggeman 2016; Tiggeman and Slater 2017). In contrast, the experiences of those who actively post (as well as view) images of their bodies online feature much less. This is surprising given the ubiquitous nature of the selfie phenomenon; a self-taken self-portrait photograph of the face or body. The data from the case studies, and in particular Chapter 5, suggest that there is a psychological consequence associated with posting images of the self for others to consume and judge in the form of comments, likes, and shares. In Chapter 5, it is evident that selfies posted online can be subject to criticism as well as praise. The practice of online body shaming – whereby other social media users post disparaging comments about a person's body – could lead to significant psychological stress, body dissatisfaction, and disordered eating. Chapter 5 suggests that selfies that are perceived to receive 'insufficient likes' might cause a young person to scrutinise their body for reasons why it did not appeal to others. In this sense, even individuals whose bodies are perceived to align with conceptions of ideal may not be immune to critique.

When social media users make 'positive' comments about a particular photograph, the implications of such comments are not necessarily positive (Chapter 5 and Chapter 6). As illustrated in Chapter 5, selfies can be a means to seek peer endorsement online and this can lead to obsessive checking behaviours. The exciting rush of a body-affirming comment is a momentary pleasure and this may distract from more meaningful human interactions. Further, with the highs come the lows – mood and affect may decrease when the frequency of positive comments inevitably slows down or when positive is not as positive as originally hoped for. The pressure to then post something new – something better – in order to achieve the next high may actually be a burden to health and wellbeing. Young people in the case studies discussed taking and posting selfies that they believed other 'people would like to see' (Chapter 5). This quote is telling, as it underlines a key feature of self-objectification; integrating the objectifying views of others into one's own belief system (Fredrickson and Roberts 1998). The selfie then can be seen as a self-objectification practice as the person posting it buys in to the idea that one's physical features are to be portrayed for (often sexual) objectification by others. Although self-objectification is typically associated with adolescent girls, the case study data showed adolescent boys also self-objectified.

Cohen and colleagues explored the link between social media selfie posts and self-objectification in a sample of 259 females (Cohen, Newton-John, and Slater 2018). Results indicated that selfie-related activity investment (i.e. time spent selecting and editing images), rather than general social networking, was associated with increased body dissatisfaction and disordered eating. This relationship was however moderated by participants' degree of self-objectification. Specifically, participants high in self-objectification and selfie investment were more likely to report bulimia symptoms. Although this was a simple correlation study, it does highlight the risks associated with posting images to please others; a practice that the case study data identified as very common.

Health and nutrition 'Insta-norms'

We have coined the term 'Insta-norms' to reflect the power of social media sites to give the impression, speedily, that marginal, fad-like health and nutrition practices are actually mainstream practices. A health and nutrition Insta-norm is when a fringe product or practice, typically dietary or fitness related, quickly trends within a social network that serves to legitimise it as normative and effective regardless of whether or not this is the case. Drawing on the case study data, we now offer examples of the ways in which health and nutrition Insta-norms come to pass.

Health and nutrition behaviour is a topic of great interest during adolescence as it is a period of significant peer comparison within a culture that emphasises attractiveness and objectification (Balentekin *et al.* 2017). It is therefore not difficult to envisage an adolescent's inclination to click a Facebook link to the next 'great' diet product or exercise regimen. The participants in the case studies described consuming 'green tea' and other purportedly healthy concoctions (see Chapter 2). As seen in Chapter 3, by clicking a health and/or nutrition link, most social media sites quickly recommend other similar articles/links of interest, so a passing interest can quickly prompt a barrage of related content. Health and nutrition content will also appear on a young person's social media feed if it has been 'liked' by a friend (Chapter 2). This can reinforce trending health and nutrition fads in two important ways. First, a further appearance on a social media feed adds to the sense that a certain product is 'everywhere' and therefore it 'must be popular and effective'. In this sense, it appears as the norm. Second, the fact that a friend who has 'liked' a certain page or article is visible to the young person provides a source of peer endorsement. As we have described, these types of peer behaviours can encourage disordered eating practices offline (Eisenberg *et al.* 2012; Erchull 2015) and the case studies suggest that they may be becoming more apparent on social media.

Diet-related Insta-norms, as behaviours promoted in youth social media activity, can be understood in terms of the concept of ethno-nutritionism. Atkinson (2011) described ethno-nutritionism as extreme or contrarian dietary norms that emerge and thrive within a subculture despite the presence of more expert knowledge outside of that culture. In terms of youth social networks, popular diet products and nutritional practices may carry greater validity than official forms of advice from the out-group (i.e. GPs, teachers, parents). For Atkinson (2011), this groupthink is driven especially by influential members of a subculture whose body types allow them to act as ambassadors or living testimonies for the benefits of a particular nutritional practice. As such, adolescent social media users who 'share' and 'like' diet products and who also conform to masculine/ feminine ideals will likely contribute forcefully to the rapid development of health and nutrition Insta-norms. When these Insta-norms are unhealthy, social networking may be an additional mechanism by which peer influence contributes to disordered eating (Meyer and Gast 2008).

Implications for addressing young people, social media, and eating disorders

Having identified a connection between social media and disordered eating, we will now discuss the implications of our analysis for research, policy, and practice.

Social media and disordered eating: Identifying causal mechanisms

Studies have consistently demonstrated significant positive associations between social media and disordered eating (Holland and Tiggemann 2016), but there is still a lack of longitudinal or experimental research in this area. Such studies are necessary to facilitate the identification of potential causal mechanisms between social media use and disordered eating. Further, most studies have focused on Facebook yet in the case studies young people reported using a variety of social media sites (e.g. Instagram and Snapchat). An important next step is to consider the impact of these newer platforms on disordered eating attitudes and behaviours.

A role for social media literacy interventions?

The case studies (Chapters 2–7) highlighted that young people may lack the skills to critically evaluate the content that they view on social media, such as targeted advertisements of dieting products and exercise regimes. The use of dieting products and dieting behaviours are strong predictors for subsequent disordered eating practices among young people (e.g. Neumark-Sztainer *et al.* 2011), so any environment that facilitates access to, normalises, or which promotes the use of such products among young people is of concern. The case studies demonstrated that young people may be encouraged to act upon the health-related material they access online (e.g. participating in exercise videos or purchasing weight loss products), which may escalate to disordered eating and exercise practices among some vulnerable individuals.

Social media literacy interventions typically aim to reduce risk factors for disordered eating by encouraging critical evaluation of the material observed on social media sites. McLean and colleagues (2017) conducted a pilot study of an intervention programme (Boost Body Confidence and Social Media Savvy intervention), comprising three 50-minute lessons that tackled issues of targeted advertising, understanding digitally manipulated images, and reducing appearance-related comparisons among peers. Encouragingly, improvements in body image and media literacy and reductions in dietary restraint were observed for the intervention group. Larger-scale and longer-term studies of social media literacy intervention programmes with more diverse groups of young people are needed to explore the wider impact that this approach might have in reducing vulnerabilities towards disordered eating behaviours.

Education and support for young people

As highlighted in Chapter 7, at present there is a disconnect between the support that is being offered to young people around social media and health and the support they would like to receive. The young people in Chapter 7 clearly identify a need for a collaborative effort between teachers, students, parents, and public health professionals in designing and developing education and support around social media and health. For example, the young people reported wanting further support about the potential negative impacts of social media. Similarly, the case studies (Chapters 2–6) highlighted the limited and unrealistic body shape and size ideals that young people are frequently exposed to on image-based social media sites. As noted earlier, this narrow definition of a 'healthy' body shape may facilitate greater body dissatisfaction and disordered eating practices among young people (Fardouly and Vartanian 2016). Within an educational setting there is a need to facilitate broader discussions around health (beyond body shape, weight, and size) that challenge some of these restricted sociocultural ideals to which young people are exposed on social media.

A school setting may be the most logical and feasible context in which to engage young people with such information, but it is essential to ensure that the material is delivered by individuals to whom young people can relate. For example, studies on literacy in schools show that many literacy interventions tend to be teacher- or peer-led, whilst others are led by trained facilitators (such as the Boost intervention; McLean *et al.* 2017). According to the wider eating disorder literature, interventions are similarly efficacious whether led by clinicians, teachers, or peers (Ciao *et al.* 2014; Stice *et al.* 2017), but programmes that incorporate face-to-face interaction are more effective than those delivered exclusively online (Stice *et al.* 2017). The case studies emphasise the value of a peer-to-peer approach, but input from adults may also be useful (e.g. around exercise regimes; dieting products) to moderate and challenge young people's perceptions of healthy behaviours. Nonetheless, it is important for teachers, parents, administrators, and researchers alike to recognise that young people are experts when it comes to their personal social media experience and involving them in the design and delivery of any intervention will be critical to its success.

A universal approach

Chapter 7 revealed that young people felt that adults (notably teachers and parents) need to be better informed about how and why young people use social media to engage with information about health, and how social media can be a useful learning resource to guide health-related behaviours. This suggests that more complex interventions may be necessary, which go beyond simply targeting young people themselves, but that also include parents, teachers, and other key stakeholders. There are several examples of complex, multi-target, disordered eating prevention programmes within the field that have been employed to good effect, and which could offer a useful framework for social media literacy focused interventions. For example, McVey and colleagues (2007) conducted an eight-month school-based universal eating disorder prevention programme (Healthy Schools-Healthy Kids), which included training for parents, teachers, school administrators, and local public health professionals, in addition to the students. The programme demonstrated positive improvements in body satisfaction and reductions in weight control behaviours among students (McVey *et al.* 2007). Whilst there are logistical and financial challenges to a universal or multi-target intervention approach, delivering a consistent message across a variety of settings is important in challenging and changing sociocultural norms.

The responsibility of social media sites

We also assert that social media sites themselves have a responsibility towards protecting the wellbeing of their users. The promotion to young people of dieting products, dieting regimes, age-inappropriate exercise schedules, and other unhealthy or harmful substances is concerning and potentially damaging to young people's health and wellbeing. The social media context can normalise unhealthy weight control behaviours and convince young people of the need to modify their body shape and size in order to meet societal ideals. There are significant challenges to regulatory control of advertising on social media spaces, but this remains another potentially effective strategy to help protect of young people (Dunlop *et al.* 2016).

Summary of key messages

- Images posted online typically reinforce the masculine muscular ideal and the feminine thin ideal. The emphasis on cultural prescriptions of normative beauty on social media sites may lead to well-established disordered eating risk factors such as body dissatisfaction, negative mood, and unorthodox dietary practices.
- Although social media hold many similarities with traditional media, certain distinct features may lead to a more powerful reinforcement of unrealistic body ideals. Specifically, the pervasiveness of mobile internet use and online connectivity dictate that idealistic depictions of beauty are ubiquitous and constant. Escaping such messages is difficult for young people as they are always connected. Further, unlike traditional magazines or movies which typically portray celebrity bodies, social media is a space where idealised images often belong to peers; increasing the personal relevance to the viewer and as such elevating the impact on mood and behaviour.
- Certain social media practices, such as posting selfies frequently and editing selfies to manipulate the image, can be associated with increased body dissatisfaction and disordered eating behaviours. This type of social networking engagement is also connected to self-objectification – a process whereby individuals learn, through interactions with others and cultural practices, to place a value on their bodies mainly as something to be sexually appreciated by others. Such 'selfie-objectification' can make those posting selfies vulnerable to the views (likes and comments) of others. In trying to satisfy the demands of the objectifying viewer, some individuals may turn to disordered eating.
- There are numerous unknowns regarding social media use and disordered eating. Much of the research evidence is correlational and specific to one or two social media sites. Little is known about the specific mechanisms by which social media might influence maladaptive eating behaviours. Social media is an ever-evolving and ever-expanding landscape and understanding its impact on disordered eating must be an ongoing endeavour.
- Multi-component interventions designed in collaboration with young people that target teachers and parents as well as adolescents should be the focus of improving social media literacy.

References

Adams, K.E., Tyler, J.M., Calogero, R., and Lee, J., 2017. Exploring the relationship between appearance-contingent self-worth and self-esteem: The roles of self-objectification and appearance anxiety. *Body Image*, 23, 176–182.

American Psychiatric Association, 2013. *Diagnostic and Statistical Manual of Mental Disorders: DSM-5 (5th Ed.)*. Arlington, VA: American Psychiatric Publishing.

Atkinson, M., 2011. Male athletes and the cult(ure) of thinness in sport. *Deviant Behavior*, 32(3), 224–256.

Bair, C.E., Kelly, N.R., Serdar, K.L., and Mazzeo, S.E., 2012. Does the Internet function like magazines? An exploration of image-focused media, eating pathology, and body dissatisfaction. *Eating Behaviors*, 13(4), 398–401.

Balantekin, K.N., Savage, J.S., Marini, M.E., and Birch, L.L., 2014. Parental encouragement of dieting promotes daughters' early dieting. *Appetite*, 80, 190–196.

Balantekin, K.N., Birch, L.L., and Savage, J.S., 2018. Family, friend, and media factors are associated with patterns of weight-control behavior among adolescent girls. *Eating and Weight Disorders – Studies on Anorexia, Bulimia and Obesity*, 1–9.

Becker, A.E., Burwell, R.A., Herzog, D.B., Hamburg, P., and Gilman, S.E., 2002. Eating behaviours and attitudes following prolonged exposure to television among ethnic Fijian adolescent girls. *British Journal of Psychiatry*, 180(6), 509–514.

Benton, C. and Karazsia, B.T., 2015. The effect of thin and muscular images on women's body satisfaction. *Body Image*, 13, 22–27.

Botta, R.A., 2003. For your health? The relationship between magazine reading and adolescents' body image and eating disturbances. *Sex Roles*, 48(9), 389–399.

Braun, V., Clarke, V., and Weate, P., 2016. Using thematic analysis in sport and exercise research. *In:* B. Smith and A. Sparkers, eds., *Routledge Handbook of Qualitative Research in Sport and Exercise*. London: Routledge, 191–205.

Brown, Z. and Tiggemann, M., 2016. Attractive celebrity and peer images on Instagram: Effect on women's mood and body image. *Body Image*, 19, 37–43.

Carrotte, E.R., Prichard, I., and Lim, M.S.C., 2017. 'Fitspiration' on social media: A content analysis of gendered images. *Journal of Medical Internet Research*, 19(3), e95.

Cheng, H.L., Tran, A.G., Miyake, E.R., and Kim, H.Y., 2017. Disordered eating among Asian American college women: A racially expanded model of objectification theory. *Journal of Counseling Psychology*, 64(2), 179.

Ciao, A.C., Loth, K., and Neumark-Sztainer, D., 2014. Preventing eating disorder pathology: Common and unique features of successful eating disorder prevention progams. *Current Psychiatry Reports*, 16(7), 453.

Cohen, R., Newton-John, T., and Slater, A., 2018. 'Selfie'-objectification: The role of selfies in self-objectification and disordered eating in young women. *Computers in Human Behavior*, 79, 68–74.

Currin, L., Schmidt, U., Treasure, J., and Jick, H., 2005. Time trends in eating disorder incidence. *British Journal of Psychiatry*, 186(2), 132–135.

Dunlop, S., Freeman, B., and Jones, S.C., 2016. Marketing to youth in the digital age: The promotion of unhealthy products and health promoting behaviours on social media. *Media and Communication*, 4(3), 35–49.

Eisenberg, M.E., Wall, M., Shim, J.J., Bruening, M., Loth, K., and Neumark-Sztainer, D. 2012. Associations between friends' disordered eating and muscle-enhancing behaviors. *Social Science and Medicine*, 75(12), 2242–2249.

Erchull, M.J., 2015. The thin ideal: A 'wrong prescription' sold to many and achievable by few. *In:* M.C. McHugh and J.C. Chrisler, eds., *The Wrong Prescription for Women: How Medicine and Media Create a 'Need' for Treatments, Drugs, and Surgery.* Santa Barbara: ABC-CLIO, 161–178.

Fardouly, J. and Vartanian, L., 2015. Negative comparisons about one's appearance mediate the relationship between Facebook usage and body image concerns. *Body Image*, 12, 82–88.

Fardouly, J. and Vartanian, L., 2016. Social media and body image concerns: Current research and future directions. *Current Opinion in Psychology*, 9, 1–5.

Fardouly, J., Diedrichs, P.C., Vartanian, L., and Halliwell, E., 2015. Social comparisons on social media: The impact of Facebook on young women's body image concerns and mood. *Body Image*, 13, 38–45.

Festinger, L., 1954. A theory of social comparison processes. *Human Relations*, 7(2), 117–140.

Field, A.E., Cheung, L., Wolf, A.M., Herzog, D.B., Gortmaker, S.L., and Colditz, G.A. 1999. Exposure to the mass media and weight concerns among girls. *Pediatrics*, 103(3), e36.

Flament, M.F., Hill, E.M., Buchholz, A., Henderson, K., Tasca, G.A., and Goldfield, G., 2012. Internalization of the thin and muscular body ideal and disordered eating in adolescence: The mediation effects of body esteem. *Body image*, 9(1), 68–75.

Fredrickson, B.L. and Roberts, T.A., 1997. Objectification theory: Toward understanding women's lived experiences and mental health risks. *Psychology of Women Quarterly*, 21, 173–206.

Goldfield, G.S., Moore, C., Henderson, K., Buchholz, A., Obeid, N., and Flament, M. F. 2010. Body dissatisfaction, dietary restraint, depression, and weight status in adolescents. *Journal of School Health*, 80(4), 186–192.

Grabe, S., Ward, L.M., and Hyde, J.S., 2008. The role of the media in body image concerns among women: A meta-analysis of experimental and correlational studies. *Psychological Bulletin*, 134(3), 460.

Griffiths, S., Murray, S.B., and Touyz, S., 2013. Disordered eating and the muscular ideal. *Journal of Eating Disorders*, 1(1), 15.

Grogan, S., 2016. *Body Image: Understanding Body Dissatisfaction in Men, Women and Children (Third Edition).* London: Routledge.

Hesse-Biber, S., Leavy, P., Quinn, C.E., and Zoino, J., 2006. The mass marketing of disordered eating and eating disorders: The social psychology of women, thinness and culture. *Women's Studies International Forum*, 29(2), 208–224.

Holland, G. and Tiggemann, M., 2016. A systematic review of the impact of the use of social networking sites on body image and disordered eating outcomes. *Body Image*, 17, 100–110.

Hummel, A.C. and Smith, A.R., 2015. Ask and you shall receive: Desire and receipt of feedback via Facebook predicts disordered eating concerns. *International Journal of Eating Disorders*, 48(4), 436–442.

Johnson, F., Pratt, M., and Wardle, J., 2012. Dietary restraint and self-regulation in eating behavior. *International Journal of Obesity*, 36(5), 665–674.

Levine, M.P. and Murnen, S.K., 2009. 'Everybody knows that mass media are/are not [pick one] a cause of eating disorders': A critical review of evidence for a causal link between media, negative body image, and disordered eating in females. *Journal of Social and Clinical Psychology*, 28(1), 9–42.

López-Guimerà, G., Levine, M.P., Sánchez-Carracedo, D., and Fauquet, J., 2010. Influence of mass media on body image and eating disordered attitudes and behaviors in females: A review of effects and processes. *Media Psychology*, 13(4), 387–416.

Loth, K.A., MacLehose, R., Bucchianeri, M., Crow, S., and Neumark-Sztainer, D., 2014. Predictors of dieting and disordered eating behaviors from adolescence to young adulthood. *Journal of Adolescent Health*, 55(5), 705–712.

Lowe, M.R. and Kral, T.V., 2006. Stress-induced eating in restrained eaters may not be caused by stress or restraint. *Appetite*, 46(1), 16–21.

McLean, S.A., Paxton, S.J., Wertheim, E.H., and Masters, J., 2015. Photoshopping the selfie: Self photo editing and photo investment are associated with body dissatisfaction in adolescent girls. *International Journal of Eating Disorders*, 48(8), 1132–1140.

McLean, S.A., Wertheim, E.H., Masters, J., and Paxton, S.J., 2017. A pilot evaluation of a social media literacy intervention to reduce risk factors for eating disorders. *International Journal of Eating Disorders*, 50(7), 847–851.

McVey, G., Tweed, S., and Blackmore, E., 2007. Healthy schools-healthy kids: A controlled evaluation of a comprehensive universal eating disorder prevention program. *Body Image*, 4, 115–136.

Mendes, V., Araújo, J., Lopes, C., and Ramos, E., 2014. Determinants of weight loss dieting among adolescents: A longitudinal analysis. *Journal of Adolescent Health*, 54(3), 360–363.

Myers, T.A. and Gast, J., 2008. The effects of peer influence on disordered eating behavior. *The Journal of School Nursing*, 24(1), 36–42.

Myers, T.A. and Crowther, J.H., 2009. Social comparison as a predictor of body dissatisfaction: A meta-analytic review. *Journal of Abnormal Psychology*, 118(4), 683–698.

Neumark-Sztainer, D., Bauer, K.W., Friend, S., Hannan, P.J., Story, M., and Berge, J.M., 2010. Family weight talk and dieting: How much do they matter for body dissatisfaction and disordered eating behaviors in adolescent girls? *Journal of Adolescent Health*, 47(3), 270–276.

Neumark-Sztainer, D., Paxton, S.J., Hannan, P.J., Haines, J., and Story, M., 2006. Does body satisfaction matter? Five-year longitudinal associations between body satisfaction and health behaviors in adolescent females and males. *Journal of Adolescent Health*, 39(2), 244–251.

Neumark-Sztainer, D., Wall, M., Guo, J., Story, M., Haines, J., and Eisenberg, M., 2006. Obesity, disordered eating, and eating disorders in a longitudinal study of adolescents: How do dieters fare 5 years later? *Journal of the American Dietetic Association*, 106(4), 559–568.

Neumark-Sztainer, D., Wall, M., Larson, N.I., Eisenberg, M.E., and Loth, K., 2011. Dieting and disordered eating behaviors from adolescence to young adulthood: Findings from a 10-year longitudinal study. *Journal of the American Dietetic Association*, 111(7), 1004–1011.

Owen, P. and Laurel-Seller, E., 2000. Weight and shape ideals: Thin is dangerously in. *Journal of Applied Social Psychology*, 30, 979–990.

Papathomas, A. and Lavallee, D., 2012. Eating disorders in sport: A call for methodological diversity. *Revista de Psicología del Deporte*, 21(2), 387–392.

Papathomas, A., 2014. A few good men: Male athlete eating disorders, medical supremacy and the silencing of a sporting minority. *In:* R. Schinke and K. McGannon, eds., *The Psychology of Sub-Culture in Sport and Physical Activity: A Critical Approach*. London: Routledge, 107–120.

Patton, G.C., Selzer, R., Coffey, C., Carline, J.B., and Wolfe, R., 1999. Onset of adolescent eating disorders: Population based cohort study over 3 years. *British Medical Journal*, 318, 765–768.

Paxton, S.J., Neumark-Sztainer, D., Hannan, P.J., and Eisenberg, M.E., 2006. Body dissatisfaction prospectively predicts depressive mood and low self-esteem in adolescent girls and boys. *Journal of Clinical Child and Adolescent Psychology*, 35(4), 539–549.

Polivy, J. and Herman, C.P., 1985. Dieting and binging. *American Psychologist*, 40, 193–210.

Rayner, K.E., Schniering, C.A., Rapee, R.M., and Hutchinson, D.M., 2013. A longitudinal investigation of perceived friend influence on adolescent girls' body dissatisfaction and disordered eating. *Journal of Clinical Child & Adolescent Psychology*, 42(5), 643–656.

Reas, D.L., Williamson, D.A., Martin, C.K., and Zucker, N.L., 2000. Duration of illness predicts outcome for bulimia nervosa: A long-term follow-up study. *International Journal of Eating Disorders*, 27(4), 428–434.

Reaves, S., Bush Hitchon, J., Park, S.Y., and Woong Yun, G., 2004. If looks could kill: Digital manipulation of fashion models. *Journal of Mass Media Ethics*, 19(1), 56–71.

Robinson, L., Prichard, I., Nikolaidis, A., Drummond, C., Drummond, M., and Tiggemann, M., 2017. Idealised media images: The effect of fitspiration imagery on body satisfaction and exercise behaviour. *Body Image*, 22, 65–71.

Shisslak, C.M., Crago, M., and Estes, L.S., 1995. The spectrum of eating disturbances. *International Journal of Eating Disorders*, 18(3), 209–219.

Silverstein, B., Perdue, L., Peterson, B., and Kelly, E., 1986. The role of the mass media in promoting a thin standard of bodily attractiveness for women. *Sex Roles*, 14(9), 519–532.

Smink, F.R.E., van Hoeken, D., and Hoek, H.W., 2012. Epidemiology of eating disorders: Incidence, prevalence and mortality rates. *Current Psychiatry Reports*, 14(4), 406–414.

Smink, F.R.E., van Hoeken, D., Oldehinkel, A.J., and Hoek, H.W., 2014. Prevalence and severity of DSM-5 eating disorders in a community cohort of adolescents. *International Journal of Eating Disorders*, 47(6), 610–619.

Smith, B. and McGannon, K.R., 2018. Developing rigor in qualitative research: Problems and opportunities within sport and exercise psychology. *International Review of Sport and Exercise Psychology*, 11(1), 101–121.

Stice, E., 1998. Modeling of eating pathology and social reinforcement of the thin-ideal predict onset of bulimic symptoms. *Behaviour Research and Therapy*, 36(10), 931–944.

Stice, E., 2001. A prospective test of the dual-pathway model of bulimic pathology: Mediating effects of dieting and negative affect. *Journal of Abnormal Psychology*, 110(1), 124.

Stice, E., 2002. Risk and maintenance factors for eating pathology: A meta-analytic review. *Psychological Bulletin*, 128(5), 825.

Stice, E., Marti, C.N., and Durant, S., 2011. Risk factors for onset of eating disorders: Evidence of multiple risk pathways from an 8-year prospective study. *Behaviour Research and Therapy*, 49(10), 622–627.

Stice, E., Presnell, K., and Spangler, D., 2002. Risk factors for binge eating onset in adolescent girls: A 2-year prospective investigation. *Health Psychology*, 21(2), 131.

Stice, E., Rhode, P., Shaw, H., and Gau, J.M., 2017. Clinician-led, peer-led and internet-delivered dissonance-based eating disorder prevention programs: Acute effectiveness of these delivery modalities. *Journal of Consulting and Clinical Psychology*, 85(9), 883–895.

Stice, E. and Whitenton, K., 2002. Risk factors for body dissatisfaction in adolescent girls: A longitudinal investigation. *Developmental Psychology*, 38(5), 669.

Striegel-Moore, R.H. and Bulik, C.M., 2007. Risk factors for eating disorders. *American Psychologist*, 62(3), 181–198.

Swami, V., 2015. Cultural influences on body size ideals: Unpacking the impact of Westernization and modernization. *European Psychologist*, 20, 44.

Thompson, J., Heinberg, L., Altabe, M., and Tantleff-Dunn, S., 1999. *Exacting Beauty: Theory, Assessment and Treatment of Body Image Disturbance*. Washington, DC: American Psychological Association.

Thompson, J.K., and Stice, E., 2001. Thin-ideal internalization: Mounting evidence for a new risk factor for body-image disturbance and eating pathology. *Current Directions in Psychological Science*, 10(5), 181–183.

Tiggemann, M. and Slater, A., 2017. Facebook and body image concern in adolescent girls: A prospective study. *International Journal of Eating Disorders*, 50(1), 80–83.

Tiggemann, M. and Slater, A., 2013. NetGirls: The Internet, Facebook, and body image concern in adolescent girls. *International Journal of Eating Disorders*, 46(6), 630–633.

Wade, T.D., Wilksch, S.M., and Lee, C., 2012. A longitudinal investigation of the impact of disordered eating on young women's quality of life. *Health Psychology*, 31(3), 352.

11 Space, place, and identity

New pressures in the lives of young people

Rachel Sandford and Thomas Quarmby

Chapter overview

This chapter examines the relationships between young people, social media, and health through an analysis of issues related to space, place, and identity. Underpinned by the work of Bourdieu and drawing on work within the field of youth geographies, we argue that the contemporary lives of young people are complex, multi-dimensional, and inter-contextual, requiring individuals to manage competing demands in both real and virtual spaces. We examine how an analysis from a broad sociological perspective can help us to better understand young people's complex engagements with social media and the resulting impacts on their negotiation and performance of identity.

Space, place, and identity

Complex social landscapes

To begin this analysis, it is important to first examine the nature and structure of social life in modern times. To do this, the broad field of sociology and specifically the social theory of Bourdieu, as well as related discussions within youth geographies, are particularly helpful. Youth geography attempts to unpack the complex spaces that young people engage with, by drawing on interdisciplinary research both within and beyond the social sciences. Importantly for this chapter, central to such research is the interrogation of children and young people's experiences of the spaces that comprise their everyday lives (both physical and virtual) and the changing nature of these spaces.

It is routinely argued that contemporary society is characterised by change and that factors such as the increased interconnectedness of peoples and the pace of evolution in human ways of life are having a significant impact on the nature of social practice and the process of identity construction (Hopkins 2010). Identity, as discussed within this chapter, is no longer perceived to be the pre-given concept of previous times, but rather a complex, multi-dimensional understanding of self that is inherently reflexive and influenced by situation and context (Blundell 2016). Changes within social structures can impact the nature of experience and thus play a key role in shaping individuals' conceptions of self. The breakdown of traditional social institutions (e.g. family, community, and religion) and changing patterns of migration and mobility, for example, are each cited as reasons for contemporary social life now being less structured and predictable than in previous generations (Allan and Crow 2001; Office for National Statistics 2017). The rapid pace of technological change adds to this complexity, changing individuals' perceptions of how we live, learn, work, and communicate (Shulman 2016). For young people 'embedded in the ebb and flow of their social worlds' (Blundell 2016, p. 8), these changes are seen to be particularly significant; leading as they do to new patterns of youth transitions, modes of communication, and agentic social action (i.e. where individuals can act independently and make free choices).

The lives of young people in contemporary Western society are complex and characterised by an increasing sense of reflexivity; meaning that individuals both shape and are shaped by their engagements with numerous social spaces (Giddens 1991; Shilling 1993). It is recognised that young people in contemporary society play an active role in the construction of spatialised identities and have the capacity to construct multi-dimensional biographies influenced by the various spaces in which they spend time. The body plays a key role in this process, being both the means by which individuals move through their social landscape and engage with social practice (Shilling 1993). As such, it is argued that bodies come to reflect the structures and practices of an individual's social world.

Concepts of space and place are important when seeking to understand and explain young people's everyday social practices, including their uses of social media, as they play a significant role in the negotiation and performance of identity. Certainly, Blundell (2016, p. 41) argues that it is important to recognise the spatiality of young people's worlds because this allows them to be positioned as social actors 'enmeshed in richly diverse social worlds rather than as separated out, disconnected individuals'. Others emphasise the importance of the relational nature of identity, reminding us that it is reliant on establishing differences and similarities between individuals and groups (Hopkins 2010). Furthermore, Anderson and Jones (2009) highlight the significance of connections between people and places in their exploration of young people's 'lifescapes' – a concept that describes how individuals are connected to places through social, spatial, and economic interactions. In a context where the nature of social life is progressively more mobile, varied, and challenging, it is perhaps easy to appreciate the challenges young people can face in navigating such complex social landscapes.

Interconnected social spaces

It is argued that one of the key challenges faced by young people in contemporary society is the interconnectedness of social spaces and the porous boundaries between these. As Hopkins (2010, p. 11) notes, 'place is now recognised as having open and permeable boundaries, shaped by complex webs of local, national and global influences, and different social and cultural flows and processes'. Literature suggests that the core social spaces for young people in contemporary society include key sites such as the family, school, peer groups, and, more recently, social media (Blundell 2016). It is noted, however, that the transient nature of these spaces means that it is possible for individuals to be simultaneously engaged in, and influenced by, the practices of different contexts at the same time e.g. discussions with peers within the school context, or connecting with friends/family via social media. This, we argue, has real implications for young people's negotiation and performance of identity.

Several authors have noted the complex nature of 'borderland' areas between interconnecting social spaces, which often require young people to navigate competing norms, values, and ideals (e.g. Somerville 2010). With the rise in the use of digital technologies, there is also an increased blurring of boundaries between real and virtual spaces (Jordan 2009). Collin *et al.* (2010) argue, for example, that young people often experience online and offline social worlds as 'mutually constituted'. There is a challenge here for identity construction, for as Chambers and Sandford (2018) note: 'Not only are individuals being required to navigate the complex, intersecting landscape of physical (actual) space, they increasingly need to do so whilst simultaneously engaging with multiple realities' (p.3).

Young people therefore not only live within localised communities that share geographical space but are also part of 'communities without propinquity' (Blundell 2016, p. 47) where interactions take place remotely and are often facilitated by technology. Appadurai (1996) argues that the global configurations of technologies that can be seen to shape social processes in contemporary society can be thought of as 'technoscapes', shaping and influencing the ways in which individuals experience technologies in their everyday lives. The rise in new technologies, and the forms of connection these support (via social media, for example) can be seen to add to this technoscape; supporting an interconnected network of virtual and physical spaces (Black *et al.* 2015). Ergler and colleagues (2016) stress the importance of theorising how technologies have changed, mediated, and affected young people's spatiality. This, they argue, better places us to learn about and understand young people's digitally mediated childhoods.

A particular area of relevance here is the degree to which digital spaces have become a fundamental part of young people's social experiences; representing taken-for-granted extensions of the physical space and becoming, as Paiva (2014) has argued, 'culturally, actual spaces' (p.2). There are some important implications here for the ways in which young people negotiate and perform identity within different interconnected socio-spatial and digitalised contexts. In the section below, we identify a theoretical framework that provides a useful lens for examining such issues in further detail.

Bourdieu's theoretical approach

As noted, it is now recognised that young people can be understood to have identities that are multi-dimensional, intercontextual, and spatialised. The subsequent discussion draws on theoretical concepts from the sociological work of Pierre Bourdieu, specifically practice, habitus, field, and capital (Bourdieu 1993, 1986, 1985, 1984) to help analyse and make sense of the social practice outlined in the case studies (Chapters 2–7). We argue that this framework offers a useful lens through which to view young people's engagements with social media and the influence of these on their conceptions of health.

Bourdieu's (1985) focus on the social world as a multi-dimensional space helps us to appreciate the intercontextual nature of social life. For Bourdieu, social processes operate within a network of social *fields*, described as partially autonomous social arenas, each with their own logic and structure to which members of the field all tacitly adhere. Fields don't stand ring-fenced but interrelate and configure in dynamic ways, thus rendering their boundaries malleable (Bourdieu and Wacquant 1992). Given that fields do not always occupy the same physical locality, it is necessary to accept the transience of field boundaries and the potential for individuals to be engaging with more than one field at a single point in time. The structure of fields is determined by the differentiation and distribution of various resources – or forms of *capital* (Bourdieu 1986).

Capital can be economic (e.g. money), cultural (e.g. qualifications), or social (e.g. status) and is valuable not in itself per se, but in the exchange value it affords an individual – for example, in changing cultural capital (e.g. educational qualifications) for economic capital (e.g. a job/wage). For Shilling (1993), the body can be viewed as a resource, functioning as a form of physical capital, with greater value being afforded to those bodies that best meet the norms, ideals, and expectations of a particular social field. An individual's capacity to acquire, consolidate, or translate capital within/across different fields determines the nature of their social practice (including their tastes and dispositions) which is then 'written into the body' via the *habitus*. Habitus is socially constructed and represents the unconscious manifestation of a range of embodied values and dispositions (Bourdieu 1984). These dispositions generate perceptions, appreciations, and practice. Importantly, habitus can be viewed through individual tastes, for example through an individual's orientation toward or preference for particular lifestyle choices. In this way, we can appreciate how social practice comes to directly influence the construction of embodied identities.

When viewed through a Bourdieusian lens we can see how the practice of the characters in the case studies (Chapters 2–7) is influenced by the values and norms embedded in their social environments and driven by the desire to acquire relevant capital that can influence (or maintain) their social position. Bourdieu's tools also facilitate an understanding of the digital landscape and allow for a focus on how 'the unequal distribution of resources may shape processes of digital inclusion for young people' (Newman *et al.* 2017, p. 565). Importantly, this theoretical framework also brings the physical body into play and helps us understand the way in which dominant ideas, norms, and values (for example around the shape, size, and appearance of bodies) come to influence individuals' tastes and dispositions. Interestingly, recent work within the physical education field has also adopted such a framework for exploring how society and culture shape young people's health (see for example, lisahunter, Smith, and emerald 2015; Wiltshire, Lee, and Williams 2017). Finally, and perhaps most importantly in the context of this chapter, a Bourdieusian framework allows for a focus on the intersections between different social spaces (real and virtual) and the processes that underpin an individual's negotiation and performance of identity within these.

Young people, social media, and space, place, and identity

This section applies the notions of field, habitus, capital, and practice to analyse the case studies (Chapters 2–7). We identify how social media sites act as specific fields (and sub-fields) to shape practice and influence young people's embodied identities in relation to health.

The field of social media

As discussed earlier, young people's social landscapes comprise a number of social fields. Each field has a specific structure and taken-for-granted logic that influences how individuals come to learn and understand the requirements of social practice in that space. With regard to issues of health, young people – such as Kelly, James, Jess, Leah, and Yaz (Chapters 2–7) – learn and acquire health-related beliefs, values, dispositions, and identities in a variety of different contexts (at home, in school, with friends) and through a variety of different pedagogic encounters (Tinning 2008). Tinning (2010) has argued the need to recognise not only 'formal' pedagogic encounters that take place in institutional sites such as schools, but also 'informal' pedagogic encounters that occur in different fields (e.g. around the table at home, in conversation with peers, reading the content of books or magazines). Social media, it could be argued, is one such pedagogic field (Bourdieu 1984); a context in which informal pedagogies (in this case about health) may be produced and reproduced. This can help to explain, for example, how engagements with social media are a means by which Kelly comes to know about diet drinks (Chapter 2), Yaz learns about the 'transformation' of the body through weight training (Chapter 3), or Leah (Chapter 4) refines her understanding of the value of particular bodies.

Bourdieu (1993) defined a field as a structured space in which beliefs and values are established and imposed on those agents within it through the various relationships and practices that occur. In the context of the case studies, this emphasises that it is not only the young people themselves, but also their family context, friendship groups, networks of connections, and, importantly, status within the broader community of social media users, that influence the nature of practice (e.g. their access to social media, what platforms they engage with, the shaping of core views/ideals etc.). Importantly, fields are also spaces of conflict and competition, structured internally in terms of power relations which locate individuals in different positions within the field (Bourdieu and Wacquant 1992). As noted, these power relations are determined by the distribution and accumulation of relevant capital (Bourdieu 1986). An individual with more capital (e.g. peer status – evidenced, perhaps, through peer endorsement or 'likes') would thus be able to secure/maintain a stronger position within the field – something that we see driving James' engagement with social media (Chapter 5). For James, having peer endorsement was a means of securing social capital and, in his mind, aiding his own personal sense of wellbeing. Something of the conflict and competition within fields, however, can also be seen within Leah's narrative (Chapter 4). While she recognises the capital (status) afforded to 'skinny girls' by posting pictures that are then 'liked', she also criticises the pressure she perceives this peer-to-peer body comparison places on others (like herself).

Negotiating practice within fields, as the case studies demonstrate, is not always easy. Although amorphous in nature and with fluid boundaries, the characteristics of social media enable it to function as a field where power is accumulated by social actors (such as Kelly, Yaz, James, Leah, and Jess). Moreover, social media can be seen to act as a distinct field of production, circulation, and exchange; rendering it an extension of the social world and part of an individual's wider lifescape (Paiva 2014). However, we should remember that the transient nature of fields and the fact that they configure in different ways for different people, means that the nature of experience is uniquely individual. While there may be shared practices, there will not always be shared impact.

Connected individuals in interconnected spaces

Social media platforms, in their various guises, are powerful tools that can connect individuals not just locally, but on a transnational scale (Papacharissi and Easton 2013). Social media collapses the boundaries through which individuals typically interact and socialise; thus, one of the most obvious forms of capital acquired within the field of social media is social capital – primarily in the form of connections with, and status among, peers. Social capital is particularly evident in Chapter 5. As James comments, ' "likes" for one of your posts is a form of peer endorsement'. James' case study highlights that on social media, social capital can be acquired by increasing connectivity (though likes) and followers, which in turn increases an individual's social status.

This is also exactly how Kelly (Chapter 2) was reported to use social media as a means of connecting with her friends (both in terms of contacting them and being contacted by them). Kelly sought to enhance her connectivity by having multiple social media accounts, and this demonstrates the perceived importance of connectivity, but also hints at the need for economic capital. For instance, easy access to economic capital (i.e. money to purchase platforms) might be needed to facilitate connections with friends. This demonstrates, perhaps, how the distribution of resources can indeed shape (or hinder) processes of digital inclusion (Newmann *et al.* 2017) and determine if/how young people can be connected. It was evident from the case study chapters that social media platforms offer young people an opportunity to accumulate and convert capital. For instance, Kelly (Chapter 2) can use social media – specifically, the group chat functions on particular platforms – to convert social capital to cultural capital. While social capital refers to an individual's stock of 'social connections' (Bourdieu 1986, p. 47), cultural capital relates to all symbolic and material goods that might give an individual a higher status in society. In this context, Kelly can draw on her online networks (her connections) to gain help and support with, for example, completing her homework.

Social capital is also relevant to the concept of resilience. Being able to draw on a stock of social capital was evident in Leah's case study (Chapter 4) as potentially useful for building resilience, since the posts circulating around Instagram had a negative impact on Leah's sense of self ('posting one picture can make someone feel insecure about themselves'). Resilience here is understood as the ability to recover from adversity and react to stressful situations (Masten 2009). Social capital, defined in a variety of different ways by various authors, has been argued to provide a useful resource for young people to draw on to access social support (connections) to overcome challenges/difficulties (e.g. Holt 2016). However, since social media collapses the boundaries through which individuals socialise, bringing fields together in virtual space, this presents an interesting dichotomy with regard to the value of these social connections and how individuals interact. Arguably, through social media young people are more connected than ever (as Kelly says, 'everyone' has social media accounts – Chapter 2). Yet, by communicating at distance, young people can also be regarded as physically more alone; in some cases, therefore, their social capital may be less effective in helping to develop resilience.

As noted, the theoretical lens of Bourdieu can help us understand how young people both shape and are shaped by their interactions with others within the field of social media (e.g. with regard to the content they access, the images they share, and the views they express). Thinking about the context of health-related social media, it is apparent why interactions between individuals can also influence their health-related practices. Fields can nurture health-related preferences, interests, and tastes (as the conscious expression of habitus) but they also mediate what social agents do in specific social, cultural, or economic contexts (Bourdieu 1984). Thus, while Kelly (Chapter 2) initially stated that she didn't choose to view images or videos related to health, these messages permeated the space to such an extent that she became resigned to the *doxa* of the field (Bourdieu 1977) and ultimately explored health-related content in the same way her friends did ('her use of social media is influenced by what everyone else does'). Arguably, those who occupy the same field, or in this case the same social media platforms, may share similar dispositions (of habitus) and reproduce the culture of their shared fields through practice (Wacquant 1992). In essence, as we grow accustomed to a new social space, our tastes and dispositions change accordingly. This perhaps reminds us that young people, like Kelly, don't fully act in and of themselves, but are influenced by the contexts in which they find themselves – that is, structure and agency are both important. Bourdieu reminds us, however, that while habitus is not fixed, it is durable. Such modification of the habitus (dispositions/tastes etc.) due to emersion in different spaces would therefore happen over time.

Spaces within spaces: the sub-fields of social media

While we may view social media as a broad field, the case study of Jess (Chapter 6) points toward the fact that different social media platforms may act as distinct sub-fields in and of themselves. Jess articulated how Instagram and Snapchat are used differently, serving different functions, by her and her friends. Her narrative suggests that Snapchat is a space to share more anecdotal stories, while Instagram serves as a space for expression and to portray a particular identity to an individual's network. There are parallels to draw here with Goffman's (1990) work on the presentation of the self, with Instagram functioning as a 'front region' and a stage on which to present a polished (managed) version of self and Snapchat representing more of a 'back region' (Bullingham and Vasconcelos 2013). Each of these sub-fields operate differently and is made distinct by the types of capital that offer the most value to the individual holders.

For Jess, for example, social capital (shared conversation) was valued more within Snapchat and physical capital ('perfect images') within Instagram. Since the taken-for-granted assumptions that help govern the practices in these sub-fields (in this case, Instagram and Snapchat) vary, and they require a different set of dispositions to act, we might consider that each social media site may encourage individuals to develop slightly different elements of habitus. These dispositions are framed by the architecture of the social media platform and therefore a young person's 'Instagram habitus' may be slightly different to their 'Snapchat habitus'. Habitus – and specifically the concepts of tastes and dispositions – are therefore particularly important in terms of analysing the case studies, especially with regard to how young people's practices shape and are shaped by engagements (their own and others') with different social media sub-fields.

The notion of individual practice both shaping and being shaped by engagement with different sub-fields is furthermore reflective of Bourdieu's notion of habitus. Rather than being deterministic, Bourdieu contended that habitus is a mediating construct shaped by the living conditions characteristic of a particular social space, whilst also operating as a 'generating principle, of classifiable practices and judgements of taste' (Laberge and Kay 2002, p. 247). The habitus is thus both structured by conditions of existence and generates particular practices in accordance with its own structure. Hence, individuals exercise agency within existing social conventions. As an example, Jess can choose to engage and express her own views within the Snapchat conversation, but is influenced both by her own tastes/values and the shared understanding of the group. This means her behaviour is socially constructed with interactions already influenced by social predispositions and rules, emanating from different social media fields.

On Instagram, the normative behaviours of the sub-field include individuals expressing and projecting their identity onto others. More specifically, individuals create narratives about their identity through images. Consider, for example, Leah's reference to the 'skinny girls with perfect hour glass figures' (Chapter 4), Yaz's affinity for body transformation videos (Chapter 3) and Jess' reference to the 'Instagram model', where you can become famous through the images that you post to social media (Chapter 6). However, when young people engage with Instagram (and other platforms), they are immediately exposed to the power relations evident within that arena. As such, young people begin to fight to acquire capital, power, and recognition in line with the rules of the field. While in the 'real' world this power and recognition may come through buying the latest designer clothes or having the latest iPhone, in the 'virtual' world, social status is recognised through the size of the social networks or the number of 'likes' and comments received. As Yaz (Chapter 3) argues, 'likes' imply 'relevance' or 'appeal'. Thus, the behaviour of accumulating connections, 'likes', or comments reflects various power relations among social actors and emerges out of the social contexts in which they find themselves (Bourdieu 1984).

In further considering power, as young people transition across different social media spaces, they are ultimately exposed to different power relations. Hence, in some sub-fields, young people can be powerless and exposed to those in charge of what Bourdieu and Passeron (1977) would label 'pedagogic authority'. In this sense, young people often uncritically believe what is communicated to them through social media platforms and consume information about health that reproduces the dominant messages about health equalling body shape. In the case of Yaz (Chapter 3), YouTube acted with pedagogic authority; identifying and suggesting videos for him to view that are reflective of the videos he has previously explored. As discussed above, the messages conveyed through these informal pedagogic encounters about body transformation, and thus health, reflect the dominant doxa of the field. That is not to say, however, that alternative perspectives on health cannot be experienced within these different arenas. For example, Yaz's friend Amy was able to recognise and reflect on these messages, demonstrate critical awareness, and identify alternative possibilities (heterodoxy) for Yaz. However, it is interesting to consider whether it was easier for Amy to adopt this critical view of Yaz's behaviour from her largely external perspective.

Performing and pausing identity in the social media field

Papacharissi and Easton (2013) have identified Instagram as a site of dramatisation and performativity, which is particularly evident in the cases of Leah (Chapter 4), James (Chapter 5), and Jess (Chapter 6). Leah's narrative depicts her friends posting pictures of their bodies; an overt display of their physical capital (Shilling 1993). Due to the doxa and pressures experienced in that space, Leah felt 'pressured' to engage in similar behaviours. In contrast, James and Jess both welcomed the opportunity to perform and display their physical capital in a space where this type of capital (in the form of bodies that conform with dominant social/cultural norms) is particularly valued. Due to the competitive nature of fields, when an individual enters a given field they will unintentionally try to extract the maximum amount of capital from every symbolic exchange (Bourdieu 1986). James and Jess are prime examples of this, whereby they both strive to convert their physical capital (their images of their appearance) into symbolic capital (in the form of likes and comments). Likes and comments on Instagram thus function as symbolic capital and shape the practices evident within that arena. For James and Jess, increasing the number of likes and comments enhances their social status.

In relation to notions of health and what is perceived to be healthy, how likes and comments function as symbolic capital in platforms such as Instagram is particularly problematic. Applying a Bourdieusian lens, the more likes and comments health-related images receive, the more the content within the image is legitimised. This, in turn, reinforces the power of the messages conveyed. If particular images portray health as synonymous with body shape, as is common within the field of physical culture (e.g. Evans *et al.* 2008), then receiving likes and comments will ultimately reinforce that as the dominant ideology. Equating health with body shape and appearance was particularly evident in Jess' case study (Chapter 6). Unlike James (Chapter 5) who drew on his social capital (connections with peers) to exchange likes with others to build his standing in the field, Jess took more drastic measures; using Photoshop to edit images of her 'ideal' self.

It would seem, then, that young people look to convert physical capital into social and symbolic capital by building social networks and accumulating followers, likes and comments based on their manufactured images. Interestingly, Papacharissi and Easton (2013) suggest that we have always tended to engage with performativity and self-editing when we present ourselves to others in real space, yet social media platforms provide an opportunity for self-editing prior to sharing. As such, they offer a 'pause' in the process of presentation; virtual space allowing for an opportunity to refine the physical self to better align with social norms. The process of self-monitoring, acknowledged as a key influence on embodied identity in contemporary society (e.g. Giddens 1991) is thus heightened through social media, which may be particularly problematic with regard to potentially harmful health-related behaviours.

The broader field of social media is therefore unique and particularly powerful since it can mobilise action both within and outside of defined spaces (Facebook, Instagram, Snapchat etc.), blurring the lines between the 'virtual' and 'real' worlds (Jordan 2009). Editing and manufacturing images that portray specific identities and perceptions of health is an example of action within that space (e.g. Jess' use of Photoshop, Chapter 6). On the other hand, action outside of that space would consist of, for example, individuals altering their diet, going to the gym, or using harmful devices to change their identity in the real world, which is then reflected back into the social media space (consider Yaz's pursuit of physical activities to increase muscle, Chapter 3, or Jess' use of the potentially harmful waist trainer, Chapter 6). Arguably, this comes down to the fact that social media platforms offer numerous arenas in which young people can engage in various actions to increase their social status; yet all form just part of their broader social landscapes.

Implications for addressing young people, social media, and space, place, and identity

This chapter has drawn on a Bourdieusian framework to offer insights into the way in which young people's use of social media shapes their practice across fields, influences their engagements with others, and impacts their negotiation/ construction of embodied identities. The discussions so far have highlighted that social media is a key field within young people's social landscapes; a space in which they exercise agency and create their own multi-dimensional biographies. However, social media is also a space that overlaps and intersects with other key fields of influence (e.g. physical culture, school, peers, etc.) which has implications for how young people negotiate and perform identity. Certainly, the increased blurring of boundaries between front and back regions (Bullingham and Vasconcelos 2013; Shulman 2016) in contemporary society and the ease with which borders between fields can be crossed suggests there may be a need to rethink our understandings of how individuals present the self in such digitally mediated landscapes. Moreover, there is potential for the borderland spaces between social media and other fields to be places of conflict or contestation; with multiple meanings, messages, ideals, and perspectives vying for prominence. As such, a key question is if, whether, and how informal pedagogic encounters within social media – in particular, concerning health-related issues – contrast with more formal pedagogic encounters (e.g. in families, schools, or sports clubs) and how best to manage potential tensions that may arise between different spaces, places, and identities.

It has been argued that young people's transitions 'within, between and across different social spaces represent a challenge for educators that has perhaps not fully been appreciated' (Chambers and Sandford, in press, n.p.). In this context, the transmission of messages within and across fields (e.g. about 'ideal' body shape, size, or appearance) can reproduce dominant norms and (mis)conceptions; with accompanying implications for an individual's health and wellbeing. This has been highlighted as a key issue within the physical education/sport literature (e.g. Fisette 2011) but some authors also note that the prevalence of engagement with social media has exacerbated this situation (Fardouly *et al.* 2015). The social practice described in the case study chapters (Chapters 2–7) illustrates this and points to the need for critical inquiry not only on the part of young people, but also for those who work with/for them, particularly with regard to promoting positive messages around health and equipping young people with the knowledge to challenge those practices that might cause harm.

Chambers and Sandford (2018) also argue that in such complex social landscapes there is a need to equip young people with 'values fluency', as a means of easing their transition between interconnecting digitally mediated social spaces. To do this, it may be necessary to meet and engage with young people in those online spaces that form such a central part of their social landscapes. Evers *et al.* (2013, p. 264), talking about sexual health communications among Australian youth, argue that it could be valuable for health professionals and educators to 'explore and create ways to listen to and engage with young people' in social media spaces; to facilitate critical discussion and debate about key issues. However, they also note that mobilising social media in this way requires sufficient resources and has implications for issues such as staff training, monitoring, and safeguarding. In addition, as this chapter has shown, there are also questions to be asked with regard to if and how adults – as individuals perceived to lack cultural and symbolic capital (consider the WhatsApp conversation about the school assembly in Chapter 7) – are able to access the field and engage in such conversations with youth.

Finally, the narratives presented appear largely homogenous, with little account taken of differences in gender, class, race, or disability. Therefore, key questions remain about how diversity is played out within the field of social media and how individuals' engagements with this space are also influenced by other aspects of their biographies. For example, how do young people with a disability engage with social media and how do they view messages about health? (How) does the lens of age, religion, class, or culture influence the way in which individuals engage with social media? How are individuals' social media experiences shaped by issues of marginalisation? Take, for instance, the example of care-experienced young people who may struggle to access social media and be under surveillance by adult carers when using it. For many care-experienced young people, use of social media may be associated with safeguarding issues and therefore restricted – or closely monitored – because of legal orders (Wilson, 2016). It would therefore be remiss to assume that all young people can access social media in the same way that their peers might. Would care-experienced youth, for example, have the same experiences (or freedoms) as Kelly, Yaz, Leah, James, or Jess (Chapters 2–6)? And, if not, would they miss out on the opportunities to build connections, acquire social capital, or work on their performance of identity? This is a good illustration, perhaps, of how social resources can shape the processes of digital inclusion or exclusion for young people in very real ways.

Building on the arguments related to homogeneity, we also need to remember that not all young people will have 'media literacy', due to varying degrees of marginalisation or disadvantage (Bird 2011). Newman *et al.* (2017, p. 559) remind us that: 'Despite the seeming ubiquity of young people's internet use, there are still many for whom access to the internet and online social networking remains inequitable and patterned by disadvantage.' The composite case studies presented in this book offer a useful initial insight into the relationships between social media, young people, and health, but we argue that further work – focused on the diverse experiences of youth – could continue to facilitate our understanding of this significant social space and the experiences of young people who engage with it.

Summary of key messages

The following key messages can be drawn from this chapter:

- Identities in contemporary times are complex, multi-dimensional, and spatialised. With digital spaces now also representing a fundamental part of young people's social experiences, there is also an increased blurring of boundaries between real and virtual space. This has some important implications for young people's negotiation and performance of online and offline identities (see also Shulman, 2016).
- The dualism of structure and agency is pertinent when considering how health is understood, portrayed, and performed in relation to social media. This dualism is helpful in understanding how individual choices pertaining to health may be shaped or constrained by wider structural forces. Hence, while young people may choose to act in certain ways when using social media platforms, these choices may be ultimately shaped by the wider social conventions and rules that govern those sites (which are, in turn, shaped by individual practice).
- Young people's dispositions, tastes, and preferences to act in certain ways are likely shaped by, and aligned with, their choices of social media platform. Thus, each social media site may encourage individuals to develop slightly different tastes or dispositions and, as such, a young person's 'Instagram habitus' may be slightly different to their 'Snapchat habitus'.
- Social media platforms, as distinct sub-fields, offer numerous opportunities for young people to accumulate and convert capital. However, when young people engage with different platforms (e.g. Instagram, Snapchat), they are immediately exposed to the power relations evident within that arena. As such, young people enter the contest to acquire relevant capital ('likes', comments, status etc.) in line with the rules of the field.
- Young people's experiences are necessarily unique, due the different ways in which fields configure in their social landscape. While these general case study narratives offer insightful perspectives on how some young people engage with social media, there is a need to further consider how different individuals may be marginalised or excluded from the digital world and, importantly, how those with different biographies view messages about health.

References

Allan, G. and Crow, G., 2001. *Families, Households and Society*. Basingstoke: Palgrave Macmillan.

Anderson, J. and Jones, K., 2009. The difference that place makes to methodology: Uncovering the 'lived space' of young people's spatial practices. *Children's Geographies*, 7, 291–303.

Appadurai, A., 1996. *Modernity at Large: Cultural Dimensions of Globalisation*. Minneapolis: University of Minnesota Press.

Bird, S.E., 2011. Are we all producers now? *Cultural Studies*, 25, 4–5.

Black, J., Castro, C., and Lin, C-C., 2015. *Youth Practices in Digital Arts and New Media: Learning in Formal and Informal Settings*. New York: Palgrave Macmillan.

Blundell, D., 2016. *Rethinking Children's Spaces and Places*. London: Bloomsbury.

Bourdieu, P., 1993. *Sociology in Question*. London: Sage.

Bourdieu, P., 1986. The forms of capital. *In:* J. Richardson, ed., *Handbook of Theory and Research for the Sociology of Education*. New York: Greenwood Press, 241–258.

Bourdieu, P., 1985. The social space and the genesis of groups. *Theory and Society*, 14.6, 723–744.

Bourdieu, P., 1984. *Distinction: A Social Critique of the Judgement of Taste*. London: Routledge & Kegan Paul.

Bourdieu, P. and Passeron, J., 1977. *Reproduction in Education, Society, and Culture*. London: Sage.

Bourdieu, P. and Wacquant, L., 1992. The purpose of reflexive sociology. *In:* P. Bourdieu and L. Wacquant, eds., *An Invitation to Reflexive Sociology*. Cambridge: Polity Press, 61–216.

Bullingham, L. and Vasconcelos, A., 2013. 'The presentation of self in the online world': Goffman and the study of online identities. *Journal of Information Science*, 39(2), 101–112.

Chambers, F. and Sandford, R., 2018. Learning to be human in a digital world: a model of values fluency education for physical education. *Sport, Education and Society*, DOI: 10.1080/13573322.2018.1515071

Collin, P., Rahilly, K., Third, A., and Richardson, I., 2010. *Literature Review: Benefits of Social Networking Services*. Sydney, Australia: CRC for Young People, Technology and Wellbeing.

Ergler, C.R., Kearns, R., Witten, K., and Porter, G., 2016. Digital methodologies and practices in children's geographies. *Children's Geographies*, 14(2), 129–140.

Evans, J., Rich, E., Davies, B., and Allwood, R., 2008. *Education, Disordered Eating and Obesity Discourse*. Abingdon: Routledge.

Evers, C., Albury, K., Byron, P., and Crawford, K., 2013. Young people, social media, social network sites and sexual health communication in Australia: 'This is Funny, You Should Watch It'. *International Journal of Communication*, 7, 263–280.

Fardouly, J. and Vartanian, L.R., 2015. Negative comparisons about one's appearance mediate the relationship between Facebook usage and body image concerns. *Body Image*, 12, 82–88.

Fisette, J.L., 2011. Exploring how girls navigate their embodied identities in physical education. *Physical Education & Sport Pedagogy*, 16(2), 179–196.

Giddens, A., 1991. *Modernity and Self-Identity*. Cambridge: Polity Press.

Goffman, E., 1990. *The Presentation of Self in Everyday Life*. London: Penguin.

Holt, N., 2016. *Positive Youth Development through Sport*. London: Routledge.

Hopkins, P. 2010. *Young People, Place and Identity*. London: Routledge.

Jordan, B., 2009. Blurring boundaries: The 'real' and the 'virtual' in hybrid spaces. *Human Organisation*, 68(2), 181–193.

Laberge, S. and Kay, J., 2002. Pierre Bourdieu's sociocultural theory and sport practice. *In:* J. Maguire and K. Young, eds., *Theory, Sport and Society*. London: JAI Press, 239–267.

lisahunter., Smith, W. and emerald, e., 2015. *Pierre Bourdieu and Physical Culture*. Oxon, England: Routledge.

Masten, A., 2009. Ordinary magic: Lessons from research on resilience in human development. *Education Canada*, 49, 28–32.

Newman, L., Browne-Yung, K., Raghavendra, P., Wood, D., and Grace, E., 2016. Applying a critical approach to investigate barriers to digital inclusion and online social networking among young people with disabilities: Digital inclusion for young people with disabilities. *Information Systems Journal*, 27, 559–588.

Office for National Statistics. 2017. *Families and households: 2017*. [Available online]: www.ons.gov.uk/peoplepopulationandcommunity/birthsdeathsandmarriages/families/bulletins/familiesandhouseholds/2017

Paiva, D., 2014. Experiencing virtual places: Insights on the geographies of sim racing. *Journal of Cultural Geography*, 32(2), 1–24.

Papacharissi, Z. and Easton, E., 2013. In the habitus of the new: Structure, agency, and the social media habitus. *In:* J. Hartley, J. Burgess, and A. Bruns, eds., *A Companion to New Media Dynamics*. London: Wiley Blackwell, 171–184.

Shilling, C., 1993. *The Body and Social Theory*. London: Sage Publications.

Shulman, D., 2016. *The Presentation of Self in Contemporary Social Life*. London: Sage Publications.

Somerville, M., 2010. A place pedagogy for global contemporaneity. *Educational Philosophy and Theory*, 42(3), 344.

Tinning, R., 2010. *Pedagogy and Human Movement: Theory, Practice, Research*. London: Routledge.

Tinning, R., 2008. Pedagogy, sport pedagogy, and the field of kinesiology. *Quest*, 60(3), 405–424.

Wacquant, L., 1992. The structure and logic of Bourdieu's sociology. *In:* P. Bourdieu, P.L. Wacquant, eds., *An Invitation to Reflexive Sociology*. Cambridge: Polity Press, 1–60.

Wilson, S., 2016. Digital technologies, children and young people's relationships and self-care. *Children's Geographies*, 14(3), 282–294.

Wiltshire, G., Lee, J., and Williams, O., 2017. Understanding the reproduction of health inequalities: Physical activity, social class and Bourdieu's habitus. *Sport, Education and Society*, iFirst Article.

12 Young people and public pedagogies of the body within social media

Emma Rich

Chapter overview

This chapter draws on work from within the field of public pedagogy to examine how young people learn about their bodies, identities, and health through social media. Drawing on the experiences of Leah (Chapter 4) and Jess (Chapter 6), I argue that young women are not only learning about body perfection codes but, in a post-feminist era, learning a series of micro-practices through which to create and modify digitised images, and generate 'value' in these social media environments. The chapter concludes by making suggestions for education programmes which include focusing on the role of affect in young people's online learning.

Public pedagogy and digital health technologies

In this chapter, I offer a public pedagogy analysis of the cases of Leah (Chapter 4) and Jess (Chapter 6). Both case chapters point to the ways in which much of what young people come to learn about their bodies, identities, and health practices is taking place through engagement with social media and other digital health technologies. There is an urgent need for critical understandings of how young people perceive, negotiate, and manage these digital environments and how this contributes to 'embodiment, selfhood and social relationships' (Lupton 2012, p. 299). I will therefore analyse the pedagogical influence (Rich and Miah 2014) of these digital technologies, identifying not only what young people are learning about 'healthy' behaviours, but how young people are learning to recognise themselves and/or others as good, healthy, active, desirable bodies in the pursuit of 'health' within these environments. In so doing, I reflect on what type of learning is taking place in these mediated environments and how these young people encounter their own bodies, subjectivities, and those of others through these digitised spaces.

Throughout this chapter I draw on work from within the field of public pedagogy (Sandlin, O'Malley, and Burdick 2011) to explore these narratives. In an earlier paper with Andy Miah, we argued for a public pedagogy approach to developing a critical understanding of digital health technologies. In outlining that framework, we expanded on the concept of 'public pedagogy', which Sandlin, O'Malley, and Burdick (2011, pp. 338–339) suggest focuses on:

> various forms, processes, and sites of education and learning occurring beyond formal schooling.... It involves learning in institutions such as museums, zoos, and libraries; in informal educational sites such as popular culture, media, commercial spaces, and the Internet; and through figures and sites of activism, including public intellectuals and grassroots social movements.

The emergence of the field of public pedagogy has presented new opportunities for theorising learning and is informed by a broad range of disciplines and literature, including curriculum studies, pedagogy, sociology, cultural studies, adult learning, lifelong learning, critical pedagogy, and feminist studies. In their comprehensive mapping of the field and review of literature spanning 1894–2010, Sandlin, O'Malley, and Burdick (2011) suggest there is a lack of theoretical and definitional clarity in relation to the conceptualisation of public pedagogy. However, whilst public pedagogy is a contested term, as the quote above suggests, there is some general consensus within the field that it comprises a focus on the kind of learning that takes place *outside* of formal schooling.

As an approach, public pedagogy offers significant potential for understanding the learning that is taking place in digital environments. It focuses on critical relationships between the educative force of a range of cultural sites in people's lives and engagement with physical practices, corporeality, and subjectivities (Rich 2011; Rich and Sandlin 2017). Whilst a body of literature has revealed how digital health technologies are the site of regulative discourses and practices, the adoption of these practices is not simple, nor can it be assumed in the broader readings of public pedagogy (see Hickey-Moody, Savage, and Windle 2010). Whilst recognising the discursive organisations of bodies is important, through our public pedagogy perspective (Rich and Miah 2014) we can also understand how users' experiences are *formed relationally*. In simple terms, what happens online is both shaped by and shapes relations with other discourses, bodies, sites, and pedagogies both within social media and beyond. Whilst an approach which focuses on dominant discourses provides some valuable insight, we have cautioned against focusing only on 'the **content** of pedagogy rather than its **relational** derivation' (Rich and Miah 2014, p. 307). Savage (2010, p. 85) warns against such 'totalizing and mythologizing' approaches to public pedagogy, which become all-encompassing and through which 'popular public pedagogies, therefore, are reduced to little more than mechanisms for exercising ideological domination'. In other words, our understanding of learning will be diminished if we fail to understand the connectedness of bodies with technologies and other bodies.

This perspective enables us to investigate the kinds of learning and education that take place via entanglements with digital technologies (see Fullagar, Rich, and Francombe-Webb 2017a, 2017b). Digital technologies form one of the many social contexts through which public pedagogies of popular culture (Sandlin, 2008, 2006; Sandlin, Burdick, and Rich 2016; Wright and Wright 2013) take place. Various scholars have begun to acknowledge how teaching and learning takes place across multiple sites/social contexts through public pedagogies, including the influence of digitised social spaces (Freishtat and Sandlin 2010; Kellner and Kim 2009). This work is necessarily multi-disciplinary and can address questions of everyday learning that take place through these social media experiences.

Whilst we have begun to explore a range of digital health technologies through this perspective of public pedagogy (Rich and Miah 2017, 2014), in this chapter I focus on the cases presented in Chapters 4 and 6, which speak specifically to social media. The proliferation of social media raises questions about the extent to which it presents new social problems and opportunities compared with other media. For example, the relationship between media and body image has long been the focus of research across a range of different disciplines (Grabe, Ward, and Hyde 2008), but we might now ask how is this experienced differently within and through social media? More recently, scholars have started to explore a range of issues related to identity, the body, and these emerging media environments (as outlined below). As will be argued, the cases in Chapters 4 and 6 are both positive, documenting the capacity for young women to be critical of imagery and health products, and concerning, because of the reification of these narrow health messages within current mediatised neoliberal postfeminist contexts.

Young people, social media, and public pedagogies

Accumulating and sharing health data/information reflects a broader expectation of individual responsibility for health (Fotopoulou and O'Riordan 2016). As such, many digital health technologies are 'instructive' and play a pedagogic role in people's everyday lives. They offer an instructional pedagogy: messages about how to monitor and regulate the body in ways that are deeply infused with a 'corporeal ethic, a socially regulative moral code' (Evans and Rich 2011, p. 365). Work within critical health education and pedagogy has examined how normalising practices are emerging across many different social sites through what is variously referred to as *body pedagogics* (Shilling 2005, 2007, 2010), *bio pedagogies* (Wright 2009; Wright and Harwood 2009), or *body pedagogies* (Evans and Davies 2004; Evans *et al.* 2008) and their specific variants. Body pedagogies are particularly pertinent to understanding the impact of learning about health and the body within digital sites, and are described as:

> Occurring over multiple sites of practice, in and outside schools, they define the significance, value and potential of the body in time, place and space, producing particular, embodied subjectivities that are essentially corporeal orientations to self and others.
>
> (Evans *et al.* 2011, p. 367)

In this earlier work with a number of other colleagues (Evans *et al.* 2009), we drew on Bernstein's notion of the pedagogic device to conceptualise the 'corporeal device'; theorising the body 'not just as a discursive construction, a conduit for the relay of messages outside itself – but as a biological body, a material relay of and for itself' (p. 393). In developing this work in relation to the way in which obesity discourse was shaping the health policies and pedagogies of schools, we revealed how schools and other institutions undertake practices to regulate bodies in relation to the norms of body perfection codes. Similarly, the narratives of Leah (Chapter 3) and Jess (Chapter 6) point towards the potential for social media to play an instructive role in their lives and through which they learn particular body perfection codes. Using these platforms forms part of their everyday day practices; for example Leah describes using them 'every second of everyday', albeit primarily for looking at sharing her friend's posts. Through their engagement with these platforms, both Leah and Jess made reference to particular body pedagogics, what Shilling (2007, p. 13) describes as:

> The central pedagogic means through which a culture seeks to transmit its main corporeal techniques, skills, dispositions and beliefs, the embodied *experiences* typically associated with acquiring or failing to acquire these attributes, and the actual *embodied changes* resulting from this process.

Thus, Leah (Chapter 4) and Jess (Chapter 6) describe working on their bodies in ways that are driven by the expectations to meet body perfection codes; maintaining their bodies through exercise, dietary practices, and styling their bodies in particular ways. Leah makes reference to the embodied experience of, in her view, failing to acquire the bodily attributes which she sees consistently being reproduced through social media imagery. As such, Leah doesn't post Instagram pictures of herself. She 'feels very self-conscious about her body' and 'wonders how people will react'. She doesn't think that her figure is 'what people want to see' and fears others might 'mock it'.

A specific feature of social media and the data it generates is the capacity for data to be shared with others, for example within social media networks, potentially leading to 'lateral surveillance' (Andrejevic 2005) of each other's bodies. This confluence of private and public spaces (Byron 2008, Papacharissi 2009) and the commercialisation of personal data raises ethical concerns about young people's privacy and the use of the data that are collected from digital health technologies. Self-presentation online presents a common point of interest for researchers of social networking sites. Through lateral surveillance of others' bodies, as young people engage with the profiles of other users, this increases opportunities for viewing images and potentially comparing their appearance to others (Kim and Chock 2015). Peer comparison and 'lateral surveillance' (Andrejevic 2005) can be a central means through which these corporeal codes are reified, through micro-practices of judgement and comparison (see Evans *et al.* 2008) which are mediated by affect and embodied experience. For some young people, the consequences of failing to meet the expectations of these corporeal codes can be incredibly harmful. Brown and Tiggeman (2016) establish that acute exposure to thin and attractive female celebrity images has an immediate negative effect on women's mood and body image. To some extent, these effects are evident in the case of Leah (Chapter 4) and I have summarised some of the key messages from this case that relate to these corporeal codes and embodied experiences.

> *Leah describes (Chapter 4) being 'really pissed' with the 'skinny girls'. She claims that it's like they just think about themselves and they don't realise how 'posting one picture can make someone feel insecure about themselves'. Leah looks at the 'skinny girls'' posts and thinks that her own figure 'is 10 times worse'. It makes Leah feel that she is 'not adequate' or 'good enough'.*

These micro-practices of comparison also occur in relation to celebrity images. For example:

> *Leah sees 'loads' of posts on Instagram of celebrities who are 'skinny' or who have 'perfect' 'hour glass figures'. But because the 'skinny girls' are 'her age' and 'she knows them', it makes her feel worse. It makes you feel like 'oh, I want to look like that'.*

Although some of the gendered norms are revealed in these particular cases (Chapter 4 and Chapter 6), further research is needed to examine the interests they serve, within particular social, cultural, and political economies. Dominant discourses pertaining to body weight, shape, and health are in this sense encoded in the regulative and instructional principles of these digital practices. They are received and articulated through the digital practices and then embodied as particular attitudes (e.g. likes) towards their own and others bodies, health, and identities. These findings raise a number of questions about the potential harms, exclusions, and impacts these behaviours might have, given the growing body of work revealing the influence of social media on body image (Cohen, Newton-John and Slater 2017; Perloff 2014). Research elsewhere reveals how, for many young people using social media, they feel pressure to lose weight, look more attractive or muscular, and to change their appearance (Pepin and Endresz 2015). Lewallen and Behm-Morawitz (2016) suggest that individuals who follow more fitness boards on the social networking site Pinterest are more likely to report intentions to engage in extreme weight loss behaviours.

In Chapter 4, the authors suggest that social media intensifies the experience of peer-to-peer body comparison. Certainly the cases of Leah (Chapter 4) and Jess (Chapter 6) speak to this, and the studies described in the above paragraphs point toward the growing evidence of intensification of negative impacts on young women's body image as a result. I would, however, go further. There is a change in the codified practices which influences the negative impacts of social media on young women's body image that involve new micro-practices, many of which are specific to the social life of data (Law and Ruppert 2013). The cases of Leah and Jess reveal micro-practices of producing, editing, and sharing images of themselves whilst also seeking out, commenting, liking, and circulating images of others. This is seen in Jess, where I have summarised some of the key messages from that chapter in relation to the micro-practices of activity and effort:

> *Jess (Chapter 6) explains how she uses social media to follow 'celebrities' ... to 'learn about their life', and she has seen them 'go from what they were to what they are now'. The 'fake celebrities' lives give Jess hope that she could become a celebrity one day. Jess is also inspired by 'something called the Instagram model'. The 'Instagram model' is where 'someone can be so famous' and 'only through a few pictures'. The 'Instagram model' is definitely something Jess could use. She just needs to post really 'polished' and 'perfect' images about her life and make sure that these posts get a lot of 'likes'.*

Within what some are describing as a postfeminist, neoliberal context (Dobson 2015), we see examples in these cases of both the pleasures, empowerment, and engagement of young women as well as surveillance, anxiety, and disaffection. Whilst efforts were made, to use Jess' words (Chapter 6) to 'perfect and polish images', these attempts to control an online identity are also subject to disciplinary practices and are shaped by corporeal codes. As Carah and Dobson (2016, p. 3) suggest 'it is precisely the social and cultural imperative to produce and to "control" images that functions as a key form of surveillance and discipline operationalised in neoliberal and postfeminist digital cultures'. Thus, on the one hand, Jess performs a subjectivity which reifies her sense of agency and control, by demonstrating her knowledge that many of these images are fake. Yet, at the same time, she continues to work on her self-representation in ways which aspire towards meeting the expectation of these narrow corporeal codes. Learning about these digital practices is both deeply affective, but also shaped by the 'political economy of gendered visual images that needs to be accounted for in analyses of identity and self-representation' (Carah and Dobson 2016, p. 3).

Jess (Chapter 6) describes learning a set of digital practices to edit photos, to pose in the right way and even to know how, when, and where to share images. These digital practices contribute to the body pedagogies or 'structures of meaning defining what the body is and ought to be' (Evans *et al.*, 2011, p. 367). The cases point towards the digital practices, social interactions, and relations which form part of these pedagogies; these are mediated body pedagogies which shape processes of differentiation and inclusion. Jess, for example, reported looking at 'fake' celebrities and trying to polish and perfect images about her life to get lots of likes, for example, using Photoshopped images to be more like the 'fake' celebrities. This process involves the production, digital editing, and maintenance of images which conform to these narrow corporeal codes. The circulation of these celebrity and peer images through mobile and other social media platforms affects other bodies (Brown and Tiggemann, 2016). Conformity to these narrow corporeal codes and the circulation of images can be understood by highlighting some of the messages from Jess' case:

> *Jess (Chapter 6) decided that her only option was 'Photoshop'. Photoshop was something she could trust and control. She could take 'a picture and edit it and actually look great'. Jess knows that this is what all the 'celebrities' and 'models' really do. So Jess spent 2 hours, in between Snapchatting Sarah, trying to get something 'perfect' to post. But although Jess was Photoshopping her photo, she didn't want it to look fake. Sometimes 'you can just tell that they are fake', 'you can see that they've Photoshopped it'. Jess wanted the real kind of fake; something that would present the 'perfect image' of the 'real her'.*

These are important insights for addressing what it is that is new about these social media imagery, given that idealised and highly gendered body imagery has long been present in all forms of media.

Carah (2014) describes social media as 'algorithmic media', given the way in which platforms' algorithms can structure content and make it visible based on predictions made about value generation. The work of Carah and Dobson (2016) is instructive here, building on this understanding of algorithmic media. In their work examining the interplay between promotion, drinking culture, and social media, they suggest that 'hot female bodies' are registered in the databases and sorted by the algorithms of social media platforms, in this instance helping viewers to 'make judgements about the desirability of locations in the nightlife' (p. 1). They go on to describe how 'images of hot female bodies generate more likes, tags and views and, over time, algorithms learn to make them more visible in the effort to translate data generated via humans' capacities to affect one another into profit' (p. 1).

In this regard, we might also begin to ask more searching questions about the way in which fitness-related images being both produced and consumed by young women form part of the political economy of media platforms. Young women like Leah (Chapter 4) and Jess (Chapter 6) are active in producing, sharing/circulating, and reviewing images as they flow affectively within social media and beyond. Similarly, Van Dijck (2013, p. 62) argues that 'popularity is not simply out there, ready to be measured: it is, rather, engineered through algorithms that prompt users to rank things, ideas or people in relation to other things, ideas or people'. The way in which these young women become 'entangled' with these algorithms (Gillespie 2014) is therefore significant in terms of how they are learning about particular digital practices. In this regard, the corporeal perfection codes are not only about meeting the expectations of developing particular bodily attributes. They are also meeting expectations about the 'correct' digital practices required to produce their digitised bodies in ways that also produce value; for example, creating and modifying an image which can affect other bodies or engage users through likes, reposting, and comments. Thus, even if the bodies of these young women met the perfection codes, there are now *additional expectations* to invest more time, knowledge, and skill into cultivating images which correspond with the correct consumption and digital practices, lifestyle, and values.

Through her engagement with these pedagogies, Jess (Chapter 6) learns how differentiation occurs as a result of these algorithmic practices:

> *Jess posted the picture to Instagram. She immediately got loads of likes. By the time she woke up, she had 200 (which is good). The photoshop had worked and she had 'faked it' well. To Jess' disappointment, however, she didn't get any comments. Comments are better than likes. BB always got loads of comments, and 'thousands, millions' of likes. Jess didn't understand what she was doing wrong. Try again she thought; try filters as well – the one's the celebs use. The filters that make you think, 'oh, that is me and I look the bomb'. Failing that, Jess said she'll have to copy Sarah and get a waist trainer.*

These experiences seem to reflect a postfeminist orientation, which in the context of neoliberalism can be described as:

> hegemonic discourses of individual choice and empowerment, freedom, self-esteem, and personal responsibility have conspired to make feminism seem second nature and therefore also unnecessary for women, especially in the Western world, where structural inequalities are increasingly viewed as personal problems that can be resolved through individual achievement.
>
> (Baer 2016, p. 20)

Jess (Chapter 6) attempts to demonstrate her individual rationality and self-awareness through not being 'fake' – yet also attempts to present herself in such a way so as to meet increasingly gendered body perfection codes. Yet, these codes are only confirmed when they are perceived to have 'value' as a result of algorithmic practices. What is perhaps unique or new about this form of media is, therefore, the role that algorithms and their associated practices (sharing, liking etc.) play in nurturing and sustaining these body pedagogies and the accompanying expectations of work required to work on one's (digitised) self.

Whilst Jess was learning the dominant corporeal codes, the 'value' of her image within these 'algorithmic media' was not sufficiently strong (i.e. not generating enough comments or likes) to demonstrate that she displayed the appropriate attributes. The work she undertakes reflects an ongoing and even relentless project of the self, reflecting a gendered subjectivity which, in a postfeminist era, is to be continually worked on and is always becoming. This learning is grounded in perpetually creating, modifying, and recreating not only 'lifestyles' but the bodies and health practices which are associated with the modified (perfected) images.

The prevailing discourses of self-improvement and optimisation implore women and girls to consume the correct digital products to work on their bodies (Rich, in press). As other users share or like these images within 'algorithmic media' such as Facebook, Instagram and so on, the social media algorithm learns the value of such images. Similarly, when fitness products/images are liked, the algorithms may make other images or products more available in users' social media feeds. Some of the young people in these chapters (for example, Chapters 2, 4, and 6) describe using products that might be regarded as unhealthy.

What is apparent from the case study chapters is the extent to which the visibility of particular bodies in the marketing of various products contributes not only to young people's consumption practices, but to the instructional and regulative body pedagogies. Sarah, Jess' (Chapter 6) friend, sent a Snapchat that conveyed her jealousy of BB: 'oh, I wish I looked like her'. Sarah was keen to find a way to look like BB. She later Snapchatted: 'I've seen on social media one of these waist trainers'. Thus as is suggested in Chapter 6, on social media, girls and young women can learn easily about harmful devices they can attempt to use to change their shape and figure. The promotion of products and services in this way reflects how 'Western media act as agents of informal education that promote and reinforce the hegemonic belief that the consumption of goods and services is the primary means of fulfilment and happiness' (Wright and Sandlin, 2017, p. 7). It is notable that a number of authors have urged scholars within the field of education to examine consumption and take it seriously as a site of learning (e.g. Sandlin and McLaren 2010a; Usher, Bryant, and Johnston 1997). Elsewhere (Rich, in press) I outline a particular theoretical approach to understanding how digital health consumption operates as pedagogy, specifically examining some of the implications for gender, power relations, and social justice across the life span. In this regard, it is useful to consider how the digital health market has potentialities and capacities through which to teach appropriate forms of health behaviour.

Negotiating products and services promoted on social media raises questions about how young people are able to navigate health knowledge online, particularly in terms of sourcing reliable and credible information on social media:

> *Jess scrolled through her Instagram home page. She found images and videos that said: 'Eating 10 kilograms of protein will help you build muscle every day'; 'The benefits of a hot and cold shower'; 'Sleep on your left side' to benefit 'your heart'; 'Smoothie that ... gets rid of the bacteria on your face ... and gives you so much energy'.*

Although wellness and lifestyle apps and devices now represent a critical mass in the digital health landscape, they are not subject to the same forms of regulation (Powell *et al.* 2014) as – for example – medical devices. Such problems may be further heightened by the proliferation of health information now available via social media, as Jess alludes to above. Whilst this knowledge will be varied and in some cases potentially helpful, concerns have been raised about the extent to which young people might be contributing to or accessing digital media that not only promote health, but which also relates to ill health or injury such as eating disorders, self-harm, or drug use. For example, concerns have been raised about 'thinspiration' images, 'thin ideal' media content (i.e. images and/or prose) that intentionally promotes weight loss, often in a manner that encourages or glorifies dangerous behaviour characteristic of eating disorders (Ghaznavi and Taylor 2015; Lewis and Arbuthnott 2012; National Eating Disorders Association 2013). Elsewhere, Tiggemann and Zaccardo (2015) describe another trend known as 'fitspiration' images that are, as described by one website, designed to motivate people to exercise and pursue a healthier lifestyle. Tiggemann and Zaccardo (2015) found that exposure to fitspiration images led to greater negative mood, body dissatisfaction, and lower appearance self-esteem. Furthermore, Lewallen and Behm-Morawitz (2016) suggest that many images which might not be allowed as *thinspiration* posts are being shared as 'fitspiration'.

Implications for addressing young people, social media, and public pedagogy

As the authors of Chapter 6 suggest, these social media platforms and their engagement are unlikely to go away anytime soon. As such, we might ask whether we can find ways to support more critical learning about and through these digital environments. Rather than make recommendations, below I signpost areas for further investigation and as potential avenues for fostering critical learning. In particular, I argue we should ask questions such as: What space is there for critical public pedagogies with a more social justice-focused orientation? How do we promote learning that will benefit young people in ways that they may feel better prepared to manage their online health identities?

The increasingly narrow definitions of acceptable bodies were alluded to in several instances in the cases. However, young people arrive at these social media practices with 'differential bodily repertoires and habits' (Ivinson 2012) and thus make sense of these images in *different ways*. For example, with reference to the performativity of the body, Leah (Chapter 4) thinks that:

> *'Skinny girls' are the worst. They post to 'find out what people think of them'. But they know that their figures are 'better than others' and they just do it for 'attention'. They caption their pictures with 'chunky monkey' or 'my thighs are big, damn it'. They say, 'oh, I'm so fat, I'm so fat' and 'they're literally like super skinny'. The 'skinny girls' are always 'saying bad stuff about their figures' and are constantly 'sticking out their pelvis' in photos, 'pretending to be fat'. The thing is, 'they clearly know their figure isn't that bad, otherwise they wouldn't have posted the picture in the first place'. Chloe, however, described how she sympathised with the skinny girls as she doesn't like being called skinny herself.*

As such, we must be cautious of essentialising such practices. The social production of gender, through the production of content and social interaction online, emerges as an assemblage through which young people learn the value of particular bodies. Earlier literature described much potential for the internet to challenge a range of inequalities including those associated with gender and normative ideals of femininity (Haraway 1991). However, the examples above reorient us towards a new set of questions pertaining to the pedagogies of algorithmic media (Carah and Dobson 2016) and the role of social media in challenging or reproducing gender norms. Whilst there are numerous examples of the potential for public pedagogies of resistance (Sandlin and Milam 2008), and reappropriation and activism through online and digital media (Kellner and Kim 2009), the experiences of the young people described in these chapters is far from straightforward.

There are already numerous examples of body image and body confidence programmes in school which are underpinned by efforts to enhance young people's media literacy. However, the examples in the case chapters suggest that young people are very aware that many media (including social media) images are fake, modified, or Photoshopped. This is particularly evident in Jess' narrative (Chapter 6):

> *BB, the latest teen celebrity, had an Instaspree (posting lots of posts in a short period of time) and everyone was Snapchatting about BB's posts. BB is one of the 'fake celebrities'. 'Most of her isn't real'. Everyone knows it's all 'money and surgery'. BB always tries to fake it though. She adds hashtags like #fit #gym #hardwork to try to trick everyone into believing that her figure has been developed through exercise. Yet, even though everyone knows BB is 'fake', girls like Jess 'still want to grow up to be like' her.*

In many ways young people are critical of these images, suggesting they already have an understanding of the damaging effects of these media imagery. For example, Leah (Chapter 4) knows it's a form of 'peer pressure' and the images are wrong, but – at the same time – she can't escape it. However, this 'rationalist' orientation is in tension with the embodied affective learning through which young people come to desire to develop bodies like those they see in these images.

As young people learn about body disaffection or the negative impact of these images, this is often in tension with the other forms of learning (e.g. via social media). In their work on critical learning in/through everyday life in a global consumer culture, Wright and Sandlin (2017) draw on the work of Jarvis (2006, 2012) concerning 'disjunctures' in learning. Wright and Sandlin (2017, p. 78) suggest that:

> When disjunctures arise in our learning/living, in this age of information, the desire to reconcile new experiences and information – which are often the result of engaging with media technologies and other public pedagogies in the first place – will often lead adults to seek resolution (new understanding and meanings) through entertainment and news media, the Internet, books, social media, film and myriad other available resources.

Drawing on this work, it can be suggested that rather than developing educational approaches steeped in notions of learning which invoke the idea of a rationalist, humanist subject, we find ways to develop understandings of the affective, embodied aspects of learning and to help young people identify disjunctures in their own learning. To draw on Ivinson (2012, p. 501), pedagogies attempting to engage young people more critically with social media may need to 'work with the gap between personal meanings and text, between *la parole* and *la langue*, embodied and formal knowledge'. In other words, it would be limiting to rely on an approach which aids young people in simply seeing 'what is really happening' (e.g. photoshopping, modifying). If this viewpoint is accepted, we need to understand how to move beyond the powerful legacies of 'the humanist project of education' (Wright and Sandlin 2017, p. 13). If we consider learning as relational (Ellsworth 2005), it is precisely in these gaps or disjunctures that we might find opportunities for young people to imagine other ways of being.

From this perspective, body knowledge and body pedagogies are contingent. Young people's bodies and their embodied knowledge become part of the very resources they draw upon to make sense of these social media material. As such, we need a better understanding of the relations between, for want of a better description, mind and body; technology and human.

Furthermore, it is important that we don't invoke polarised understandings. Young people are learning within and across these different social sites simultaneously (see Fullagar, Rich, and Francombe-Webb 2017a, 2017b). This posthumanistic perspective of learning could, potentially, open up further spaces for understanding experiences such as those of Leah (Chapter 4) and Jess (Chapter 6), but to explore alternatives. The co-implication of bodies, subjectivities, and algorithms also becomes pedagogically significant as these young women learn what is of 'value'. Examining the relationship between social media platforms and corporations might, for example, be the subject of a critical pedagogy which helps young women understand the micro-politics within which work on the self takes place.

Summary of key messages

- The cases described in Chapters 4 (Leah) and 6 (Jess) point to the complexities of social media and the need to avoid technological determinism; social media is neither inherently oppressive nor empowering. Their experiences *are both positive* – documenting the capacity for young women to be critical of imagery and health products – *and concerning* – because of the reification of these narrow health messages within current mediatised neoliberal postfeminist contexts.
- Dominant discourses pertaining to body weight, shape, and health are encoded in the regulative and instructional principles of the digital practices young women might be learning online. Social media can further intensify the 'body image' pressures generated through media norms.

- New codified practices are emerging in digital environments which come to influence the negative impacts of social media on young women's body image. Specifically, these involve new micro-practices related to the social life of data. There is therefore pressure to meet expectations about the 'correct' digital practices required to produce their digitised bodies that are of 'value'.
- Traditional media literacy programmes might be necessary, but not sufficient in helping young people to navigate these digital landscapes. Educational programmes will need to focus on the embodied affective learning through which young people come to desire to develop bodies like those they see in these images.

References

Andrejevic, M., 2005. The work of watching one another: Lateral surveillance, risk, and governance. *Surveillance*, 479–497.

Baer, H., 2016. Redoing feminism: Digital activism, body politics, and neoliberalism. *Feminist Media Studies*, 16(1), 17–34.

Brown, Z. and Tiggemann, M. (2016) Attractive celebrity and peer images on Instagram: Effect on women's mood and body image. *Body Image*, 19, 37–43.

Byron, T., 2008. Safer children in a digital world: The report of the Byron Review. Available from: http://webarchive.nationalarchives.gov.uk/20130401151715/www.education.gov.uk/publications/eOrderingDownload/00334-2008.pdf

Carah, N., 2014. Curators of databases: Circulating images, managing attention and making value on social media. *Media International Australia*, 150, 137–142.

Carah, N. and Dobson, A., 2016. Algorithmic hotness: Young women's 'promotion' and 'reconnaissance' work via social media body images. *Social Media + Society*, October–December, 1–10.

Cohen, R., Newton-John, T., and Slater, A., 2017. The relationship between *Facebook* and *Instagram* appearance-focused activities and body image concerns in young women. *Body Image*, 23, 183–187.

Dobson, A.S., 2015. *Postfeminist Digital Cultures: Femininity, Social Media, and Self-Representation*. New York, NY: Palgrave Macmillan.

Evans, J. and Davies, B., 2004. The embodiment of consciousness: Bernstein, health and schooling. *In:* J. Evans, B. Davies, and J. Wright, eds., *Body Knowledge and Control*. London: Routledge, 207–218.

Evans, J., Davies, B., and Rich, E., 2008. The class and cultural functions of obesity discourse: Our latter day child saving movement. *International Studies in Sociology of Education*, 18(2), 117–132.

Evans, J., Rich, E., Davies, B., and Allwood, R., 2008. *Education, Disordered Eating and Obesity Discourse*. London: Routledge.

Evans, J. and Rich, E., 2011. Body policies and body pedagogies: Child matters in totally pedagogised schools? *Journal of Education Policy*, 26(3), 361–379.

Fotopoulou, A. and O'Riordan, K., 2016. Training to self-care: Fitness tracking, bio-pedagogy and the healthy consumer. *Health Sociology Review*, 26(1), 1–15.

Freishtat, R.L. and Sandlin, J.A., 2010. Facebook as public pedagogy: A critical examination of learning, community, and consumption. *In*: T.T. Kidd and J. Keengew, eds.,

Adult Learning in the Digital Age: Perspectives on Online Technologies and Out-comes. Hershey, PA: Information Sciences Reference, 148–162.

Fullagar, S., Rich, E., and Francombe-Webb, J., 2017a. New kinds of (ab)normal? Public pedagogies, affect and youth mental health in the digital age. *Social Sciences,* 6(3), 99.

Fullagar, S., Rich, E., and Francombe-Webb, J., 2017b. Youth mental health in the digital age: Understanding public pedagogies as affective arrangements. *Social Sciences.*

Ghaznavi, J. and Taylor, L.D., 2015. Bones, body parts and sex appeal. An analysis of #thinspiration images on popular social media. *Body Image,* 14, 54–61.

Grabe, S., Ward, L.M., and Hyde, J.S., 2008. The role of the media in body image concerns among women: A meta-analysis of experimental and correlational studies. *Psychological Bulletin,* 134(3), 460–476.

Haraway, D.J., 1991. *A Cyborg Manifesto: Science, Technology, and Socialist-Feminism in the Late Twentieth Century;* Routledge: New York, NY, USA.

Hickey-Moody, A., Savage, G.C., and Windle, J., 2010. Pedagogy write large: Public, popular and cultural pedagogies in motion. *Critical Studies in Education,* 51(3), 227–236.

Ivinson, G., 2012. The body and pedagogy: Beyond absent, moving bodies in pedagogic practice. *British Journal of Sociology of Education,* 33(4), 489–506.

Jarrett, K., 2014. The relevance of 'women's work': Social reproduction and immaterial labor in digital media. *Television & New Media,* 15(1), 14–29.

Jarvis, P., 2012. Learning from everyday life. *HSSRP,* 1(2), 1–20.

Jarvis, P., 2006. *Towards a Comprehensive Theory of Human Learning.* London: Routledge.

Kellner, D. and Kim, G., 2009. YouTube, critical pedagogy, and media activism: An articulation. *In:* R. Hammer and D. Kellner, eds., *Media/Cultural Studies: Critical Approaches.* New York, NY: Peter Lang, 615–636.

Kim, J.W. and Chock, T.M., 2015. Body image 2.0: Associations between social grooming on Facebook and body image concerns. *Computers in Human Behaviour,* 48, 331–339.

Law, J. and Ruppert, E., 2013. The social life of methods: Devices. *Journal of Cultural Economy,* 6(3), 229–240.

Lewallen, J. and Behm-Morawitz, E., 2016. Pinterest or Thinterest?: Social comparison and body image on social media. *Social Media + Society,* January–March 1–9.

Lewis, S.P. and Arbuthnott, A.E., 2012. Searching for thinspiration: The nature of interest searches for pro-eating disorder websites. *Cyberpsychology Behaviour Social Network,* 15(4), 200–204.

Lupton, D., 2012. M-health and health promotion: The digital cyborg and surveillance society. *Social Theory & Health,* 3, 229–244.

Papacharissi, Z., 2009. The virtual geographies of social networks: A comparative analysis of Facebook, LinkedIn and ASmallWorld. *New Media & Society,* 11(1/2), 199–220.

Pepin, G. and Endresz, N., 2015. Facebook, Instagram, Pinterest and co.: Body image and social media. *Journal of Eating disorders,* 2015, 3(Suppl 1), O22.

Perloff, R.M., 2014. Social media effects on young women's body image concerns: Theoretical perspectives. *Sex Roles,* 71 (11–12), 363–377.

Powell, A.C., Landman, A.B., and Bates, D.W., 2014, In search of a few good apps. *Journal of The American Medical Association,* 311(18), 1851–1852.

Rich, E., in press. Making gender and motherhood through pedagogies of digital health and fitness consumption 'soon it made us more active as a family'. *In:* D. Parry, C. Johnson, and S. Fullagar, eds., *Digital Dilemmas: Transforming Gender Identities and Power Relations in Everyday Life.* Palgrave Macmillan.

Rich, E. and Miah, A., 2014. Understanding digital health as public pedagogy: A critical framework. *Societies*, 4, 296–315.

Rich, E. and Miah, A., 2017. Mobile, wearable and ingestible health technologies: Towards a critical research agenda. *Health Sociology Review*, 26(1), 84–97.

Rich, E. and Sandlin, J.A., 2017. Physical cultural studies and public pedagogies. *In:* M. Silk, H. Thorpe, and D. Andrews, eds., *Routledge Handbook of Physical Cultural Studies.* London, UK: Routledge, 549–557.

Sandlin, J.A., 2008. Consumption, adult learning, and adult education: Envisioning a pedagogy of consumption. *Convergence*, 41, 47–62.

Sandlin, J.A., 2006. Lifestyle magazines as informal consumer education: Evidence from a qualitative analysis of budget living. *Journal of Consumer Education*, 23, 1–13.

Sandlin, J.A. and McLaren, P., 2010. *Critical Pedagogies of Consumption: Living and Learning in the Shadow of the 'Shopocalypse'.* Oxon and New York: Routledge.

Sandlin, J.A., Burdick, J., and Rich, E., 2016. Problematizing public engagement within public pedagogy research and practice. *Discourse: Studies in the Cultural Politics of Education*, 38, 823–835.

Sandlin, J.A. and Milam, J.L., 2008. 'Mixing pop [culture] and politics': Cultural resistance, culture jamming, and anti-consumption activism as critical public pedagogy. *Curriculum Inquiry*, 38, 323–350.

Sandlin, J.A., O'Malley, M.P., and Burdick, J., 2011. Mapping the complexity of public pedagogy scholarship: 1894–2010. *Review of Educational Research*, 81, 338–375.

Sandlin, J.A., Wright, R.R., and Clark, C., 2013. Reexamining theories of adult learning and adult development through the lenses of public pedagogy. *Adult Education Quarterly*, 63, 3–23.

Savage, G., 2010. Problematizing 'public pedagogy' in educational research. *In:* A.J. Sandlin, B.D. Shultz, and J. Burdick, eds., *Handbook of Public Pedagogy.* New York, NY: Routledge, 103–115.

Savage, G.C., 2014. Chasing the phantoms of public pedagogy: Political, popular and concrete publics. *In:* J. Burdick, J.A., Sandlin, and M.P. O'Malley, eds., *Problematizing Public Pedagogy.* New York, NY: Routledge, 79–90.

Tiggemann, M. and Zaccardo, M., 2015. 'Exercise to be fit, not skinny': The effect of fitspiration imagery on women's body image. *Body Image*, 15, 61–67.

Usher, R., Bryant, I., and Johnston, R., 1997. *Adult Education and the Postmodern Challenge.* London: Routledge.

Van Dijck, J., 2013. *The Culture of Connectivity: A Critical History of Social Media.* Oxford, UK: Oxford University Press.

Wright, J., 2009. Biopower, bio pedagogies and the obesity epidemic. *In:* J. Wright and V. Harwood, eds., *Biopolitics and the Obesity Epidemic.* London: Routledge, 1–15.

Wright, J. and Harwood, V., 2009. *Biopolitics and the 'Obesity Epidemic'.* London: Routledge.

Wright, R.R. and Sandlin, J.A., 2017. (Critical) learning in/ through everyday life in a global consumer culture. *International Journal of Lifelong Education*, 1–2, 77–94.

Wright, R.R. and Wright, G. L., 2013. Investigating sci-fi and horror for critical adult education and teacher education: Learning international perspectives and valuing the 'other'. *International Journal of Innovative Learning and Leadership*, 1, 6–12.

13 The role of social media in developing young people's health literacy

Dean A. Dudley, Penny Van Bergen,
Anne McMaugh, and Erin Mackenzie

Chapter overview

In this chapter, the notion of health literacy is explored in the context of adolescents learning about health. Up until fairly recently, the concept of health literacy has been driven mainly by health care models and has specifically targeted adult populations. This chapter uses the case studies (Chapters 2–7) provided to explore an alternative way of discussing and promoting health literacy and in ways that draw on the perspectives of young people and their frequent engagement with social media in a digital age.

What is health literacy?

A plethora of literature supports the notion that future patterns of adult health are established during childhood and adolescence (Due *et al.* 2011; Sawyer *et al.* 2012; Suppli *et al.* 2012). There is also strong evidence to suggest that the longitudinal impact of health in adolescence may continue throughout adulthood and into old age (World Health Organization 2014). It is, therefore, critically important to influence health behaviours at an early age. According to the United Nations (2015), the cost of inaction in the early years is immense. Millions will continue to die from preventable diseases and rising health care costs will continue to plunge millions of people into poverty, with non-communicable diseases (NCD) alone expected to cost low- and middle-income nations more than US$7,000,000,000,000 in the next 15 years. By better understanding the risks and drivers of adolescent health, we are better able to promote and inform health and wellbeing behaviours across the lifespan.

It is important to recognise that adolescents may not interact with public health information in the same way as adults. One critical difference is in the ways in which adolescents make extensive use of social media to interact with their friends, share ideas, seek help, and access new information (Swist *et al.* 2015; Third *et al.* 2017, 2014). Recent research suggests that more than half of adolescents now use social media daily (Mackenzie 2018), and this has possible implications for both knowledge and behaviour. In this chapter we explore the potential benefits and risks of social media use for adolescent health literacy. We begin by considering adolescent public health more broadly. We then describe health literacy in adolescence, and apply this model to social media use in order to consider the case of Yaz presented in Chapter 3. We conclude by considering the implications for how health literacy and social media use interact to produce health-related behaviour change.

Adolescents and public health

Given the impact of adolescent health on lifetime health outcomes, a number of public health programmes and initiatives have highlighted the importance of changing the health-related behaviours of young people. These include the United Nations Sustainable Development Goals programme (United Nations 2015) that focuses on ensuring healthy lives and the promotion of wellbeing for all. A significant proportion of adolescents residing in developed/high-income nations (especially as socio-economic disparity widens) fail to meet many of the recommended healthy behaviour guidelines set by their respective government agencies (i.e. daily consumption of fruit and vegetables, sleep requirements, physical activity participation) (Elgar *et al.* 2015) and many also suffer from a growing prevalence of mental health illnesses (Steel *et al.* 2014). This is despite most adolescents in these settings having access to the systems and knowledge that can develop the recommended health-related behaviours and lead to immediate, sustained, and long-term effect on health and wellbeing.

While public health programmes and initiatives are increasingly highlighting the importance of targeting young people, these efforts have also often focused on specific risks, rather than broader health literacies. For example, strategies that address NCD risk have tended to focus on secondary prevention and treatment to reduce the conversion of risk to disease (Lobstein, Baur, and Uauy 2004; National Research Council 2009). While these approaches reduce morbidity and mortality, their impact on adolescents is limited: especially considering the tracking evidence that shows adolescence is a sensitive period in which both normative and maladaptive health-related behaviours shape future trajectories (Sawyer *et al.* 2012). Part of this sensitivity involves brain changes that create conditions for heightened receptivity to health messages and social norms. These changes are linked to the social embedding of health-related behaviours and the biological changes that occur during and beyond adolescence (Sawyer *et al.* 2012). Primary prevention/health promotion efforts, therefore, offer the unique potential to promote the development of positive health-related behaviours, consequently contributing to reducing the exponential growth of the global NCD burden (Balbus *et al.* 2013).

Developmental theorists have recognised adolescence as a critical period of both psychological and biological development (Viner *et al.* 2012). During adolescence, rapid development of the central nervous system and other biological systems interact with an individual's social development and capacity to build peer relationships. This facilitates new health-related behaviours that allow many important transitions for an individual to function as a productive adult

(Viner *et al.* 2012). The prefrontal cortex, the site of executive control functions, influences planning, emotional regulation, decision-making, and self-awareness, and is one of the brain regions that undergoes the most protracted development during adolescence (Sawyer *et al.* 2012). This explains the somewhat perplexing phenomenon that although there is substantial improvement in self-control from childhood to adulthood, young adolescents can at times be surprisingly immature in practices of risk-aversion and planning. Compounding this possibility is evidence that the limbic system, which governs reward processing, appetite, and pleasure seeking, develops earlier in adolescence than the prefrontal cortex (Casey *et al.* 2008). Thus, adolescents may have a tendency to make poor decisions not because they are less intellectually capable, but because they are more affected than adults by exciting or stressful situations. This is especially likely to be the case when making decisions in the presence of peers, and particularly on social media.

Understanding the implications of the nature and timing of adolescent neuro-cognitive maturation on health promotion efforts for young people has been somewhat limited, despite the proliferation of adolescent development theories in educational contexts. It has been argued, therefore, that building health literacy in young people could be one way to make use of what is already known and to develop a workable approach to more effective forms of public health promotion.

Healthy literacy in adolescence

The human right to education has become a necessary means for public health intervention during the early years of development, especially in adolescence (WHO 2008). Much work has been accomplished in ensuring that most young people around the world are educated at least to the level of lower secondary education (i.e. up to 15 years of age) (UNESCO 2017). The most basic foundation of the education of human beings is the ability to understand, read, write, and calculate. These essential life skills translate into the broader term of 'literacy'. As these skills are the foundational skills required in order to exercise the right to engage in education, literacy can be considered as an essential right (UNESCO 2013). Literacy is, therefore, not only a tool but an essential step in the achievement of many of the United Nations Sustainable Development Goals that are endorsed by the World Health Organization (United Nations 2015).

Over the last 50 years, theories of 'literacy' have evolved from those focused solely on changes in an individual to more complex views encompassing the broader social contexts (i.e. the 'literate society') (Dudley *et al.* 2017). There has been an evolution from viewing literacy as a simple process of acquiring basic skills, to using these skills in ways that develop the capacity for social awareness and critical reflection as a basis for personal and social change (Street 2006). The body of literature linking health and literacy is rigorous and the relationship between literacy skills and a variety of health outcomes has been established (Berkman *et al.* 2011).

Health literacy as a discipline-derived literacy can be traced back to the 1970s (Simonds 1974) and was formally documented by Kickbusch and Nutbeam (1998) in the World Health Organization's Health Promotion Glossary. In this document it was defined as:

> cognitive and social skills which determine the motivation and ability of individuals to gain access to, understand, and use information in ways which promote and maintain good health.
>
> (World Health Organization 1998, p. 10)

According to Rudd (2017), health literacy has emerged as an important consideration and variable for investigation for health researchers, practitioners, and policy makers. In turn, it is becoming evident that health literacy acts as a determinant of health in the empirical literature (Rudd 2017). This too has implications for issues of equity as well as for health disparities within many countries. The fact that literacy can now be linked to many health outcomes means it has become the focus of an increasing number of research studies, as well as the stimulus for institutional and governmental policy in many developed countries (Berkman *et al.* 2011).

The term health literacy is now commonly used to evaluate the capabilities of people to access and act upon relevant health-related information and processes (and the systems that manage them). New questions have now arisen in the context of educative and pedagogical perspectives of health literacy (Peralta *et al.* 2017). This need for an educative focus in health literacy is partly driven by concern surrounding the influence of information about health that is readily available via social media. A recent article by Peralta *et al.* (2017) proposed a conceptual framework for health literacy in adolescence as a process of identifying and elaborating relevant interrelated elements. They included existing theoretical and empirical work on adult health literacy, media literacy, whole school health research and practice, capability development and practice, critical health literacy, and young people.

Peralta *et al.* (2017) argued that many social determinants contribute to an individual's health across their lifetime. Many of these social determinants have particular importance during adolescence. For example, safe and supportive families and schools and positive and supportive peers are crucial to helping young people develop to their full potential and attain the best health in their transition to adulthood (Peralta *et al.* 2017). Given the overwhelming acknowledgement that social determinants contribute to an individual's health, it would be remiss not to investigate the role that social media might play during this critical life phase, especially in the development of health literacy.

Young people, social media, and health literacy

In this section the relationship between health literacy and social media is analysed by drawing on the existing literature and evidence from the case study chapters (Chapters 2–7). We examine (i) the opportunities for growth, (ii) cognitive risks and opportunities, and (iii) social risks and opportunities.

Opportunities for growth

From a health literacy perspective, social environments (including those in the virtual space like social media) should create opportunities to enhance young people's autonomy, motivation, decision-making capabilities, peer connections, and emotional control (Peralta *et al.* 2017). They do this by providing learning experiences both within and outside the controlled school environments (Peralta *et al.* 2017). These social environment opportunities allow for an exploration into the social determinants of health, and how specific social environments may influence an individual's health and the health of others with whom they interact. An exploration into social environments can also provide insights into how opportunities exist for adolescents to build on their existing knowledge, and whether these social environments prompt adolescents to reflect on the importance of this knowledge in their own lives and the lives of others. This is a key functioning part of health literacy for adolescents. In other words, adolescents should become health literate for themselves and in relation to others, while understanding the perspectives of others and of the collective. This capability cannot be developed, however, if health information is acquired in isolation or without opportunities for adolescents to apply new health information and skills across their everyday lives (Peralta *et al.* 2017).

A recent article by Roberts *et al.* (2017) suggests that social media could serve as a means of connecting people and organisations around important areas of common discourse (notably health). This is because social media platforms offer opportunities for quick and in-depth dialogue with a diverse and plentiful array of stakeholders from anywhere in the world (Roberts *et al.* 2017). Across the case study chapters (Chapters 2–7), the narratives demonstrated that young people were interacting with a diverse range of health-related stakeholders, either directly or indirectly, and were able to engage in dialogue quickly. In this sense, the opportunities to interact with a range of stakeholders is an example of how social media could support the growth of young people and the development of health literacy. Yet, as an increasing number of people (especially young people) receive their news and health information online via social media platforms (Swist *et al.* 2015), it is important to ensure content delivered through online media is not only accessible but also accurate. Swist *et al.* (2015) also argue that the effective incorporation of social media into existing health literacy programmes depends on the use of best evidence health literacy strategies, which include (but are not limited to) the use of plain language techniques.

Cognitive risks and opportunities

Related to the conceptual model of health literacy outlined above is research from the cognitive sciences that examines media literacy in a digital age.

Information about health and wellbeing can be shared widely online and public health campaigners and government departments frequently use online channels to promote messages about health policies and programmes (Australian Government Department of Health 2015). Therefore, and building on the discussions around growth, there are plentiful opportunities to connect people and organisations around important areas of health discourse. Yet the constant availability of information online is a double-edged sword, with information from non-credible sources and commercial ventures often equally prominent. Adolescents who use social media frequently may, therefore, be at particular risk of poor decision-making about their health for two main reasons. For example, there was evidence of adolescents' access to commercial information and poor decision-making in Chapter 2.

Evidence suggests that young people who lack expertise in a domain – for example, pre-existing health literacy – are at heightened risk of conceptual misunderstanding when they seek or find information online (see Poundstone 2016). When searching for health information on Google, for example, prior knowledge about various health phenomena will guide the formation of search cues. Prior knowledge will also guide the interpretation of information encountered passively via social media by underpinning critical thinking skills and whether or not adolescents are able to effectively evaluate the veracity of the information that is presented to them. Those without expertise are at heightened risk of being attracted to information that is scientifically invalid or inappropriate (Poundstone 2016), and are less likely to critique the information they find (Willingham 2007). We see this demonstrated in the case study narrative of Yaz (Chapter 3), with his uncritical use of bodybuilding videos and health-related information. The problem of a lack of critical awareness can be exacerbated on social media, where adolescents become unwitting and passive consumers of a range of populist articles and ideas, company product placement, sponsored news items, and other unregulated information about health and wellbeing that is shared with them. There was also evidence across the case study chapters (Chapters 2–7) of young people's exposure to this type of social media health-related content.

Evidence suggests that poor decision-making also relates to the range of cognitive heuristics, or 'mental short-cuts' (see Strough, Karns, and Schlosnagle 2011; Weber and Johnson 2009). The 'mental short-cuts' taken by adolescents mean that they may be less able to critically assess the health-related information they are presented with on social media (Riva *et al.* 2015). This is the case even where prior knowledge is present, and it therefore poses a particular problem to the ways in which adolescents' access and then act up on the health-related information available on social media. The problem is furthered on social media as each social media post is shared transiently and adolescents access information quickly. For example, Yaz (Chapter 2) finds the content online to be highly accessible and quick to use: 'You can look in "two minutes"'. As he is accessing information quickly it can be suggested that he is taking 'mental short cuts' and he is likely to be less able to critically evaluate that content. The interaction of

Yaz's pre-existing cognitive beliefs with the design and expediency of social media creates the perfect context for rapid influence of social media health-related content on his health and wellbeing.

One of the most common 'mental short cuts' that people use when sharing information is a short cut known as 'social loafing'. In social loafing, people intrinsically tend to reduce their effort when collaborating with others, as they assume that others will do more cognitive work for them. In a social media environment, therefore, adolescents may assume that the person sharing the information with them will already have assessed it critically and so they do not need to. There was evidence of this in Chapters 2 and 6, where Kelly and Jess each engaged with health-related content promoted by peers, commercial parties, and/or celebrities. Social loafing is made more problematic again by the presence of a second mental short cut, the familiarity bias. According to the familiarity bias, people who are not critically attending to the material that they are reading often estimate the probability that a particular piece of information is true based purely on their exposure to the idea (Begg, Anas, and Farinacci 1992; Moons, Mackie, and Garcia-Marques 2009). According to this reasoning, an idea that is heard often enough 'must be true'. Thus, Kelly's (Chapter 2) frequent exposure to FitTea advertisements leads her to view this product as healthy, because 'they must be really popular'. The workout videos frequently promoted to Yaz (Chapter 3) also leads him to begin to believe in health-related discourses such as 'no pain, no gain'. Neither Kelly or Yaz seem aware that the posts shown on social media are determined by algorithms (see Chapters 2 and 3), with the friends, products, and services that a user has previously interacted with being more likely to be seen again.

The problematic issues related to adolescents' decision-making skills when using social media are further reflected in the literature reporting variation between adolescents in their abilities to critically evaluate sources of information online. For example, Kiili *et al.* (2018) presented 426 Finnish adolescent students with an online academic health resource and an online commercial health resource. One-quarter of students performed particularly well, demonstrating a strong ability to assess the credibility of both the academic and the commercial source. Almost half of the adolescents (48.6%) however did not, and one in five (19%) failed to recognise any potential for commercial bias. This evidence suggests that adolescents require considerable support in learning how to determine the credibility of information.

Importantly, developing critical health literacy should equip young people with the skills to better assess the health information they encounter via social media. This is a case of the strong getting stronger: while social media offers a vehicle for learning about health, some degree of health literacy is needed in order to learn effectively and to rule out incorrect information. This critical literacy is particularly pertinent given that information presented via social media is typically considered only briefly, such as in the case of Yaz (Chapter 3). It is therefore critical that young people both take the time to evaluate the sources that they encounter on social media, and have the critical literacy skills to do so.

Social risks and opportunities

The above section on the cognitive risks and opportunities of developing health literacy in a digital age highlights the importance of both expertise and deliberate efforts in assessing information online. While this is true for all online sources of information, social media is also inherently social; providing a context in which social norms can be both enacted and established. Social networking and information sharing are ubiquitous in adolescent peer relationships (Swist *et al.* 2015; Third *et al.* 2017), and it is critical to understand how the social aspects of these relationships influence health outcomes. Sociologists have furthermore long proposed that social change originates from cohorts of young people with common experiences (Bolton *et al.* 2013). Social media may therefore be leading to large-scale changes in social norms and behaviours of young people in domains including health.

For several decades, theories of normative beliefs and perceived social norms have suggested a pathway through which beliefs influence behaviour. While the association between such beliefs and subsequent behaviours is not exact (Fishbein and Ajzen 1975), normative beliefs and perception of social norms have been implicated in a host of behavioural and health-related outcomes; for example, within college students' alcohol abuse (Prentice and Miller 1996), smoking behaviours (Grube, Morgan, and McGee 1986), and childhood aggressive behaviours (Huesmann and Guerra 1997). More recently, online and social media contexts have been scrutinised as a mechanism through which broader social networks and access to sources of information can influence the beliefs-behaviour relationship. For example, body dissatisfaction beliefs were linked to the tendency of college men and women to internalise media representations of thinness and attractiveness and becoming preoccupied by weight, dieting, and eating restraint (Dye 2016). Internalisation of unrealistic body ideals in video games also led to lower body satisfaction in men (Sylvia *et al.* 2014). This evidence suggests pathways from prior normative beliefs about the body towards internalisation of social norms, and also the acquisition of new beliefs or social norms after being presented with idealised images or exemplars.

In the case of Yaz and his friend Amy (Chapter 3), pre-existing normative beliefs about body image and body dissatisfaction may be linked to a preoccupation with searching for related information online. The social media sites Yaz and Amy visit could also be presenting them with social norms about male or female body types. For Amy, it was evident that she has benefited from engaging with the social media campaign, This Girl Can. The campaign was designed to alter adolescents' and young women's pre-existing beliefs about body type and present new social norms about the body and exercise. Amy benefited from this campaign as she reported that her engagement in physical activity increased through altering her perception of the type of body that was required to engage in physical activity. For example, Amy appeared to have discovered a new social norm in the campaign that showed her 'it is ok to look like an absolute slob when I run'. In contrast to Amy, Yaz (Chapter 3) did not find sources of information about exercise relevant to young men his age. In effect, Yaz's pre-existing normative beliefs about the ideal or desirable male body were not challenged as they were for Amy, so his preoccupation with searching for information related to body building increased his vulnerability to 'helpful' search algorithms; these algorithms likely recommended content related to his initial search for exercises and thus reinforced his pre-existing beliefs of a muscular body type. In particular, Yaz engaged with the YouTube videos that may have been harmful to his health, because the exercise regimes met his pre-existing beliefs and the sites appeared to 'guarantee' success in achieving his perception of an ideal body type.

Chapter 3 also demonstrates clear differences in the ways in which young people engage with health-related information. In contrast to Yaz, Amy was able to critique Yaz's use of videos from YouTube and she was sceptical about the content that he was engaging with. This finding can be supported by evidence that suggests that not all adolescents are equally vulnerable to internalisation of projected norms or ideals or the resulting negative effects (Diviani *et al.* 2015). As we argued earlier in this chapter, health and media literacy may serve a protective function, enabling adolescents to make sensible and well-reasoned judgements about media or health-related information. A review of existing research indicates that low levels of health literacy lead to the application of unhelpful and erroneous criteria to evaluate the quality of online health information (Diviani *et al.* 2016), indicating that Yaz may have had a lower level of health literacy. Mclean *et al.* (2016) also found that media literacy could decrease the vulnerability of adolescents to media images of the thin ideal appearance, suggesting that Amy may have a higher level of media literacy. Although we do not know Amy's level of health or media literacy, the case study in Chapter 3 indicates that Amy is more aware of the health consequences of certain behaviours and more aware of the capacity of social media to 'pressure' Yaz.

Implications for addressing young people, social media, and health literacy

There is little doubt that social media platforms are becoming a powerful educational resource that exist in our digital age. They appear to be a medium in which young people are prepared to utilise health information and form decisions regarding their subsequent health behaviours. The evidence is less clear, however, about whether they are effective in supporting health literacy that leads to sustained health-change behaviours. At best, social media is a *double-edged sword* where health literacy can be challenged or reinforced. We argue that the development of adolescents' health literacy should be a central focus of health promotion initiatives and this can be achieved via peer support, as well as support from adults.

Peer support (friends and acquaintances)

The importance of peer relationships to adolescents indicates that peers will have a significant influence on social norms and health literacy. As adolescents obtain health information from a range of interpersonal (friends, family), as well as media (online) socialisation agents (Paek, Reber, and Lariscy 2011), peers with better health literacy may have the capacity to offset the negative images that adolescents are exposed to online. As shown in Chapter 3, Yaz's friend Amy demonstrates an understanding that the fitness videos to which Yaz is exposed are not appropriate for him, and that his adherence to the fitness regime may have negative consequences for his health and wellbeing. Thus, if adolescents have well-developed health literacy, they may be able recognise when their peers' uptake of social media-driven norms is problematic. Interventions to increase adolescent health literacy may be a useful way to offset the effects of exposure to problematic online content. Indeed, peer-led interventions have been successful in influencing behaviours that have direct implications for health, including substance use, diet, eating, and exercise (Crosnoe and McNeely 2008).

Whilst increased health literacy may allow peers to act as the first identifier of a problem, adolescents also need to be supported to confront any problematic behaviour or seek help to support a friend or acquaintance in need. Although adolescents find it easier to get help for others than themselves (Raviv *et al.* 2000), it may also be difficult for adolescents to offer help to their friends. For example, Byrne *et al.* (2016) found that adolescents would avoid offering support to friends if they felt that the issue was a private matter, or if they were unsure of how to help. Further, Latkin and Knowlton (2015) recommend that social network-based interventions between peers would benefit from explicit communication training to heighten (or change) social norms. Indeed, the way in which peers offer assistance may be problematic without explicit support and training. For example, research on adolescents' responses to peers with mental health problems suggests that most do not respond in a way that will facilitate getting the help required. While they are likely to offer social support, many report that they would not assist their peer to seek adult assistance (Byrne *et al.* 2015; Coles *et al.* 2006; Mason *et al.* 2015).

Adult support (teachers and parents)

Adolescents are most likely to turn to friends for support (Bullot *et al.* 2017; Crystal *et al.* 2008). Yet other relationships are also implicated in the provision of support, and these relationships offer important pathways for improving adolescent health literacy online and offline. For example, parents' level of eHealth literacy (the ability to access quality health information on the internet) is positively related to adolescents' eHealth literacy (Chang *et al.* 2015). Teachers also have a key role to play in improving adolescents' health literacy (Skopelja *et al.* 2008; Tappe and Galer-Unti 2001). For example, evaluation of the Dove campaign (see Chapter 3) in one-off classroom interventions has shown that teacher-led interventions as opposed to researcher-led interventions had greater effects on the targeted health behaviour post intervention (Diedrichs *et al.* 2015). We also saw in Chapter 7 that Yaz appeared to be aware that teachers could offer him and his peers information to support their critical use of social media and need for health information. Taken together, it appears that adolescent relationships with their peers, parents, and teachers can support them to improve their health literacy, and reduce the impact of exposure to online content via social media.

According to Goodyear *et al.* (2018a), young people are tethered to their digital devices and social media relationships. This presents an obligation for schools to educate young people to use social media to support health literacy that can, in turn, generate positive health behaviours across the life course. Access to social media, like education, is now viewed as a right and as essential for youth wellbeing (Third *et al.* 2014). By understanding the health risks and opportunities that result from young people's access to social media, a new health literacy imperative now exists. Teachers and other adults responsible for educating young people about their health and wellbeing are confronted by the complexity that health literacy poses. However, interventions on social networking platforms support the notion that health behaviour changes can be effective in general but that effects are moderated by age and gender (Yang 2013). Given that effect sizes in these interventions are greater in young people, developing combined media/health literacy interventions during compulsory years of schooling is a worthwhile venture.

In acknowledging the contribution adults play in developing the media and health literacy of young people, adults should also engage in ongoing conversations with young people to ensure they act in ways that respect young people's media and health literacy needs (Goodyear *et al.* 2018a). In summary, we agree with Goodyear *et al.* (2018b) that adults in these roles need to be sufficiently media and health literate to protect young people from harm but also promote positive health behaviour norms and change when needed.

Summary of key messages

- Developing health literacy in young people is an important construct that should be considered in the context of engagement with social media.
- Normative beliefs shape adolescents' searches for information and their interactions on social media. In turn, social media use can reinforce social norms.
- Social media use offers potential benefits for adolescents' health literacy, with greater availability of information and with the potential for shared dialogue and positive normative beliefs that enhance healthy behaviours.
- Social media use may also place some aspects of adolescents' health at risk, with unregulated information and unhealthy social norms also easily shared.
- Interventions that target peer, parent, and teacher support may provide opportunities for improving adolescent health literacy to reduce negative impacts of exposure to online content.

Acknowledgement

The authors wish to recognise the contribution of Dr Louisa Peralta from the University of Sydney for her insight on some of the current literature pertaining to health literacy.

References

Australian Government Department of Health. 2015. *Social Media: How the Department is Using Social Media Channels.* Retrieved 20 January 2018 from www.health.gov.au/internet/main/publishing.nsf/Content/social-media-channels.

Balbus, J.M., Barouki, R., Birnbaum, L.S., Etzel, R.A., Gluckman, P.D., Grandjean, P., and Jensen, G.K., 2013. Early-life prevention of non-communicable diseases. *Lancet,* 381(9860).

Begg, I., Anas, A., and Farinacci, S., 1992. Dissociation of processes in belief: Source recollection, statement familiarity, and the illusion of truth. *Journal of Experimental Psychology: General,* 121, 446–458.

Berkman, N.D., Sheridan, S.L., Donahue, K.E., Halpern, D.J., Viera, A., Crotty, K., … and Tant, E., 2011. Health literacy interventions and outcomes: An updated systematic review. *Evidence Report/Technology Assessment,* 199, 1–941.

Bolton, R.N., Parasuraman, A., Hoefnagels, A., Migchels, N., Kabadayi, S., Gruber, T., … and Solnet, D., 2013. Understanding Generation Y and their use of social media: A review and research agenda. *Journal of Service Management,* 24(3), 245–267.

Bullot, A., Cave, L., Fildes, J., Hall, S., and Plummer, J., 2017. *Mission Australia's 2017 Youth Survey Report.* Mission Australia.

Byrne, S., Swords, L., and Nixon, E., 2015. Mental health literacy and help-giving responses in Irish adolescents. *Journal of Adolescent Research,* 30(4), 477–500.

Casey, B.J., Jones, R.M., and Hare, T.A., 2008. The adolescent brain. *Annals of the New York Academy of Sciences,* 1124(1), 111–126.

Chang, F.-C., Chiu, C.-H., Chen, P.-H., Miao, N.-F., Lee, C.-M., Chiang, J.-T., and Pan, Y.-C., 2015. Relationship between parental and adolescent ehealth literacy and online health information seeking in Taiwan. *Cyberpsychology, Behavior, and Social Networking,* 18(10), 618–624.

Coles, M.E., Ravid, A., Gibb, B., George-Denn, D., Bronstein, L.R., and McLeod, S., 2016. Adolescent mental health literacy: Young people's knowledge of depression and social anxiety disorder. *Journal of Adolescent Health,* 58(1), 57–62.

Crosnoe, R. and McNeely, C., 2008. Peer relations, adolescent behavior, and public health research and practice. *Family and Community Health,* 31, S71–S80.

Crystal, D.S., Kakinuma, M., DeBell, M., Azuma, H., and Miyashita, T., 2008. Who helps you? Self and other sources of support among youth in Japan and the USA. *International Journal of Behavioral Development,* 32(6), 496–508.

Diedrichs, P.C., Atkinson, M.J., Steer, R.J., Garbett, K.M., Rumsey, N., and Halliwell, E., 2015. Effectiveness of a brief school-based body image intervention 'Dove Confident Me: Single Session' when delivered by teachers and researchers: Results from a cluster randomised controlled trial. *Behaviour Research and Therapy,* 74, 94–104.

Diviani, N., van den Putte, B., Giani, S., and van Weert, J.C., 2015. Low health literacy and evaluation of online health information: A systematic review of the literature. *Journal of Medical Internet Research,* 17(5).

Dudley, D., Cairney, J., Wainwright, N., Kriellaars, D., and Mitchell, D., 2017. Critical considerations for physical literacy policy in public health, recreation, sport, and education agencies. *Quest*, 69(4), 436–452.

Due, P., Krølner, R., Rasmussen, M., Andersen, A., Trab Damsgaard, M., Graham, H., and Holstein, B.E., 2011. Pathways and mechanisms in adolescence contribute to adult health inequalities. *Scandinavian Journal of Public Health*, 39(6_suppl), 62–78.

Dye, H., 2016. Does internalizing society and media messages cause body dissatisfaction, in turn causing disordered eating? *Journal of Evidence-Informed Social Work*, 13(2), 217–227.

Elgar, F.J., Pförtner, T.K., Moor, I., De Clercq, B., Stevens, G.W., and Currie, C., 2015. Socioeconomic inequalities in adolescent health 2002–2010: A time-series analysis of 34 countries participating in the health behaviour in school-aged children study. *The Lancet*, 385(9982), 2088–2095.

Fishbein, M. and Ajzen, I., 1975. *Belief, Attitude, Intention, and Behavior: An Introduction to Theory and Research*. Reading, MA: Addison-Wesley.

Goodyear, V.A, Armour, K.M., and Wood, H., 2018a. Young people and their engagement with health-related social media: new perspectives. *Sport, Education and Society*, iFirst.

Goodyear, V.A, Armour, K.M., and Wood, H., 2018b. *The Impact of Social Media on Young People's Health and Wellbeing: Evidence, Guidelines and Actions*. Birmingham UK: University of Birmingham.

Grube, J.W., Morgan, M., and McGee, S.T., 1986. Attitudes and normative beliefs as predictors of smoking intentions and behaviours: A test of three models. *British Journal of Social Psychology*, 25, 81–93.

Huesmann, L.R. and Guerra, N.G., 1997. Children's normative beliefs about aggression and aggressive behavior. *Journal of Personality and Social Psychology*, 72(2), 408–419.

Kickbusch, I. and Nutbeam, D., 1998. Health promotion glossary. *Geneva: World Health Organization*, 14, 1–36.

Kiili, C., Leu, D.J., Marttunen, M., Hautala, J., and Leppänen, P.H.T., 2018. Exploring early adolescents' evaluation of academic and commercial online resources related to health. *Reading and Writing*, 31(3), 533–557.

Lobstein, T., Baur, L., and Uauy, R., 2004. Obesity in children and young people: A crisis in public health. *Obesity Reviews*, 5(s1), 4–85.

Mackenzie, E., 2018. *Support Seeking in Early and Middle Adolescent Girls: An Exploratory Study of Online Support Seeking and Mental Health*. Unpublished doctoral dissertation: Macquarie University, Sydney, Australia.

McLean, S.A., Paxton, S.J., and Wertheim, E. H., 2016. Does media literacy mitigate risk for reduced body satisfaction following exposure to thin-ideal media? *Journal of Youth and Adolescence*, 45(8), 1678–1695.

Mason, R.J., Hart, L.M., Rossetto, A., and Jorm, A.F., 2015. Quality and predictors of adolescents' first aid intentions and actions towards a peer with a mental health problem. *Psychiatry Research*, 228(1), 31–38.

Mikkilä, V., Räsänen, L., Raitakari, O.T., Pietinen, P., and Viikari, J., 2004. Longitudinal changes in diet from childhood into adulthood with respect to risk of cardiovascular diseases: The cardiovascular risk in young Finns study. *European Journal of Clinical Nutrition*, 58(7), 1038–1045.

Moons, W.G., Mackie, D.M., and Garcia-Marques, T., 2009. The impact of repetition-induced familiarity on agreement with weak and strong arguments. *Journal of Personality and Social Psychology*, 96, 32–44.

National Research Council. 2009. *Preventing Mental, Emotional, and Behavioral Disorders among Young People: Progress and Possibilities.* Washington, DC: National Academies Press.

Paek, H.-J., Reber, B.H., and Lariscy, R.W., 2011. Roles of interpersonal and media socialization agents in adolescent self-reported health literacy: A health socialization perspective. *Health Education Research*, 26(1), 131–149.

Peralta, L., Rowling, L., Samdal, O., Hipkins, R., and Dudley, D., 2017. Conceptualising a new approach to adolescent health literacy. *Health Education Journal*, 76(7), 787–801.

Poundstone. 2016. *Head in the Cloud: Why Knowing Things Still Matters When Facts Are so Easy to Look Up.* New York: Little, Brown and Company.

Prentice, D.A. and Miller, D.T., 1996. Pluralistic ignorance and the perpetuation of social norms by unwitting actors. *Advances in Experimental Social Psychology*, 28, 161–209.

Raviv, A., Raviv, A., Vago-Gefen, I., and Fink, A. S., 2009. The personal service gap: Factors affecting adolescents' willingness to seek help. *Journal of Adolescence*, 32(3), 483–499.

Riva, S., Antonietti, A., Iannello, P., and Pravettoni, G., 2015. What are judgment skills in health literacy? A psycho-cognitive perspective of judgment and decision-making research. *Patient Preference Adherence*, 23, 1677–1686.

Roberts, M., Callahan, L., and O'Leary, C., 2017. Social media: A path to health literacy. *Information Services & Use*, 37(2), 177–187.

Rudd, R., 2017. Health Literacy: Insights and Issues. *In:* R.A. Logan and E.R. Siegel, eds., *Health Literacy: New Directions in Research, Theory and Practice*, 240, 60.

Sawyer, S.M., Afifi, R.A., Bearinger, L.H., Blakemore, S.J., Dick, B., Ezeh, A.C., and Patton, G.C., 2012. Adolescence: A foundation for future health. *The Lancet*, 379(9826), 1630–1640.

Simonds, S.K., 1974. Health education as social policy. *Health Education Monographs*, 2(1_suppl), 1–10.

Skopelja, E.N., Whipple, E.C., and Richwine, P., 2008. Reaching and teaching teens: Adolescent health literacy and the internet. *Journal of Consumer Health on the Internet*, 12(2), 105–118.

Steel, Z., Marnane, C., Iranpour, C., Chey, T., Jackson, J.W., Patel, V., and Silove, D., 2014. The global prevalence of common mental disorders: a systematic review and meta-analysis 1980–2013. *International Journal of Epidemiology*, 43(2), 476–493.

Street, B. 2006. Understanding and defining literacy. *Background Paper for EFA Global Monitoring Report.*

Strough, J., Karns, T.E., and Schlosnagle, L., 2011. Decision-making heuristics and biases across the lifespan. *Annals of the New York Academy of Schiences*, 1235, 57–74.

Suppli, C.H., Due, P., Henriksen, P.W., Rayce, S.L.B., Holstein, B.E., and Rasmussen, M., 2012. Low vigorous physical activity at ages 15, 19 and 27: Childhood socio-economic position modifies the tracking pattern. *The European Journal of Public Health*, 23(1), 19–24.

Swist, T., Collin, P., McCormack, J., and Third, A., 2015. *Social Media and the Well-being of Children and Young People: A Literature Review.* Perth, WA: Prepared for the Commissioner for Children and Young People, Western Australia.

Sylvia, Z., King, T.K., and Morse, B.J., 2014. Virtual ideals: The effect of video game play on male body image. *Computers in Human Behavior*, 37, 183–188.

Tappe, M.K. and Galer-Unti, R.A., 2001. Health educators' role in promoting health literacy and advocacy for the 21st century. *Journal of School Health*, 71(10), 477–482.

Third, A., Bellerose, D., Oliveira, J.D.D., Lala, G., and Theakstone, G., 2017. *Young and Online: Children's Perspectives on Life in the Digital Age.* Sydney: Western Sydney University.

Third, A., Bellerose, D., Dawkins, U., Keltie, E., and Pihl, K., 2014. *Children's Rights in the Digital Age: A Download from Children Around the World.* Melbourne: Young and Well Cooperative Research Centre.

UNESCO, 2017. *Global Education Monitoring Report 2017/18 – Accountability in Education: Meeting Our Commitments.* UNESCO Press: Geneva.

United Nations, 2015. *Transforming Our World: The 2030 Agenda for Sustainable Development – Sustainable Development knowledge platform.* Retrieved from https://sustainabledevelopment.un.org/post2015/transformingourworld on 23 November 2017.

United Nations Education, Scientific, and Cultural Organization., 2013. *Paper on Literacy from a Right to Education Perspective.* Retrieved from http://unesdoc.unesco.org/images/0022/002214/221427e.pdf on 10 November 2017.

Viner, R.M., Ozer, E.M., Denny, S., Marmot, M., Resnick, M., Fatusi, A., and Currie, C., 2012. Adolescence and the social determinants of health. *The Lancet*, 379(9826), 1641–1652.

Weber, E.U. and Johnson, E.J., 2009. Mindful judgment and decision making. *Annual Review of Psychology*, 60, 53–85.

Willingham, D., 2007. Critical thinking: Why is it so hard to teach? *American Educator*, 8, 9–19.

World Health Organization, 2014. *International Classification of Functioning, Disability and Health.* Geneva, Switzerland: Author. Retrieved from www.who.int/classifications/icf/en/ on 20 November 2017.

WHO Commission on Social Determinants of Health, and World Health Organization, 2008. *Closing the Gap in a Generation: Health Equity through Action on the Social Determinants of Health: Commission on Social Determinants of Health Final Report.* World Health Organization.

Yang, Q., 2017. Are social networking sites making health behavior change interventions more effective? A meta-analytic review. *Journal of Health Communication*, 22(3), 223–233.

14 The role of internet memes in shaping young people's health-related social media interactions

Ashley Casey

Chapter overview

The chapter considers Dawkins' (1976) conceptualisation of memes as culture units that spread from brain to brain through the process of imitation. Internet memes offer an alternative perspective through which to view young people's health-related social media encounters. Drawing on the case studies (Chapters 2–7), I explore these data-rich narratives through three themes: (i) genre of participation; (ii) algorithms not people as transmitters of culture; and (iii) adults (teachers and parents). In so doing, I argue for the need for new spaces in which young people and adults can begin to explore their digital futures.

Memes and internet memes

Memes

Memes are not new to health and physical education (HPE). Richard Tinning (2014, 2012) has twice employed memes to open our eyes to the possibility of alternative considerations of established crises in HPE. He did this first by arguing that the cultural practice of physical education in schools and universities has endured despite an adamant belief that the subject is broken and dangerously close to extinction (Kirk 2010; Tinning 2012). Second, Tinning (2014) argued that the accelerating virulence of the so-called 'obesity crisis' serves the goals of physical activity and health organisations but often fails to protect or promote the health of young people. In short, Tinning (2014) argued that certain ideas become prominent while others wither and die.

In making these memetic arguments, Tinning (2014, 2012) drew heavily on the work of the evolutionary biologist Richard Dawkins (1976) who first coined the term 'meme'. He also drew on the work of other memetic theorists such as Lynch (1996) and Blackmore (1999), to argue that both the teaching of physical education and the obesity crisis were ideas that were being replicated in the cultural discourses of HPE and wider society.

Dawkins (1976) argued that the most significant 'thing' that made humankind unusual was culture. No other species, he argued, has or shares culture. No other species replicates and transmits cultural practices as do humans; nor does any other species have cultural replicators, for example, stories, books, songs. In seeking a term to encapsulate his idea of cultural transmission or cultural replication, Dawkins (1976) used the term memes. Dawkins (1976) argued that memes are living structures that have permanence and penetrance in the cultural environment. In other words, 'memes are units of culture that spread from person to person through copying or imitation' (Shifman 2014, p. 2). Likening memes to genes, and placing them in their own meme pool, Dawkins (2006, p. 249) suggested that:

> Just as genes propagate themselves in the gene pool by leaping from body to body via sperms or eggs, so memes propagate themselves in the meme pool by leaping from brain to brain via a process which, in the broadest sense, can be called imitation.

Scholars have argued (c.f. Blackmore 1999; Dawkins 2006, 1976; Dennett 1991; Zappavigna 2012) that memes survive and replicate because of a combination of (a) longevity, which in most cases is very short – at least in evolutionary terms, (b) fecundity, the rate at which a meme replicates itself in a culture, and (c) copying-fidelity, the amenability of an idea to transmission. In other words, some ideas endure such as the example of the obesity crisis or – in the context of this book – the fallibility of young people in the digital world and the need for adults to repeatedly tell them what is best for them. Some memes are passed down not only between generations but also across cultures, while others (like the idea that world is flat) cease to be replicated and subsequently die.

Given their potential to spread, Dawkins (1976, p. 207) argued that memes should be regarded as 'living structures' and that 'when you plant a fertile meme in my mind you literally parasitize my brain, turning it into a vehicle for the meme's propagation in just the same way as a virus may parasitize the genetic mechanism of a host cell'. Thus it is easy to understand why traditional ideas about parenting have endured; for example, 'spare the rod, spoil the child'. Indeed, and as I will argue later in this chapter, it is unsurprising that parents today use different 'rods' (i.e. the confiscation of mobile devices) to avoid having their child(ren) spoilt (by social media).

Internet memes

The application of the term memes to phenomena on the internet was not made until the 1990s. Writing in *Wired*, Mike Godwin (1994, no page number) argued that 'it's time for net dwellers to make a conscious effort to control the kinds of memes they create'. In an interview in the same magazine, Dawkins (see Solon 2013) argued that the term internet meme was a hijacking of the original idea of a meme, because an idea proliferated through the internet does not mutate by random chance but through human creativity. Consequently, an internet meme has come to represent the internet-fuelled propagation of items such as videos, jokes, rumours, and websites (Shifman 2014). Recent internet memes include the ice bucket challenge[1] and Success Kid.[2]

In her consideration of how young people are living in and with networked publics,[3] boyd (2014, p. 211) suggested that 'today's teens – regardless of their personal levels of participation – are coming of age in an era defined by easy access to information and mediated communication'. In short, boyd (2014, p. 211) argued that 'the rise of mobile devices is … taking the already wide-spread notion of being "always on" to new levels'. Perhaps most worryingly, from the perspective of this book, is the understanding that while this digital viral world is being rapidly populated by young people, memetic ideas about parenting and teaching are proving slower to change. Indeed, Jenkins *et al.* (2016, p. viii) argued that while young people are inimitably placed to effect social change – due to their position as 'lead adaptors of mobile, social and gaming media' – they face 'conditions of oppression … in making their perspectives heard and appreciated'. Significantly, whilst we supposedly live in a participation culture, young people's ability to create and share content across the internet is purposefully disconnected from their capacity to influence the governance of the same networks (Jenkins, Ito, and boyd 2016). In other words, while young people are trailblazing social spaces, their voices are being deliberately excluded from the decision-making processes.

The cultural background in which memes originally emerged is very different from the digitised and wireless world of today. Blackmore (1999) argued that the digitising of information has served to increase the copy-fidelity of any potential meme or, as Zappavigna (2012, p. 100) argued, 'the internet … facilitates fast meme production'. At a time when information and the attention people pay to it are seen as being valuable (Shifman 2014) the meme has become a 'cultural touchstone' (Milner 2016) by which an idea or event is judged. When Dawkins (1976) wrote his thesis it would have almost impossible to imagine the virality of information in the digital world. In 1976 it might have taken three days for 40,000 people to receive a news event through print media, word of mouth, telephone, and/or letter (Nahon and Hemsley 2013). Today three minutes might suffice. News had limited sources and conduits in 1976. Now everyone has the potential to be a newscaster, particularly through social media.

The networked publics where young people live full-time are filled with internet memes (boyd 2014). An internet meme was defined by Shifman (2014 p. 41) as:

> Group of digital items sharing common characteristics of content, form, and/or stance, which were created with awareness of each other, and were circulated, imitated, and/ or transformed via the Internet by many users.

If you consider the 'things' that travel your own online networks you will recognise similarities in content, form, and stance. In fact, the array of complex algorithms created by social media sites (Tuten and Solomon 2012) go a long way to guaranteeing that this is the case. These algorithms are not created randomly or haphazardly but are created by social media sites to contribute to the small conversations that personify contemporary media (Milner 2016). They can be regarded as the '*lingua franca*'[4] for digital participation (Milner 2016, p. 7).

Dawkins (2006) conceptualised memes as competitive. He posited that memes would compete for our time and some would live and some would die; 'the human brain, and the body that controls it, cannot do more than a few things at once. If a meme is to dominate the attention of a human brain, it must do so at the expense of "rival" memes' (p. 255). Only by dominating the attention of a human brain/body long enough to be shared can a meme hope to survive. Indeed, only when this type of sharing occurs across a network or culture can ideas truly be considered memetic. The idea of deliberately creating memes via algorithms (as I will discuss later) goes against Dawkins' idea that they would be competitive. In a world where only the fittest survives, this algorithmic practice suggests that algorithmically enhanced memes are being created. What concerns me is the potential harmful impact that these well-financed and well-supported internet memes might have on young people's health-related social media encounters.

Shifman (2014) contends that while the spread of internet memes occurs at a micro level – for example through the social networks of young people – the impact of such memes can be experienced at a macro level; for example, by challenging and changing the thought processes and subsequent actions of young people as a collective. Internet memes are 'digital snippets that can make a joke, make a point, or make a connection … they are the linguistic, image, audio, and video texts created, circulated, and transformed by countless cultural participants across vast networks and collectives' (Milner 2016, p. 1). If, as Dennett (2017, p. 206 original emphasis) suggests, memes are '*a way of behaving* (roughly) that can be copied' then both information or misinformation might be 'transmitted or saved under the [belief or] mistaken presumption that it is valuable'. Like counterfeit money, which is saved and later spent, misinformation regarding health might be used to the potential detriment of the young person/persons concerned.

Internet memes are also ways of belonging and being on the inside. They are badges or insignia often only recognisable by other, likeminded individuals and groups. Zappavigna (2012, p. 101) argues that it is not the explicit nature of an internet meme that increases one's 'cool quotient' but knowing how to use the meme in the correct context. Internet memes are as much about the inside joke as they are about the funny picture/message (Zappavigna 2012). It is the way internet users 'wield this inside joke' that indicates whether they are 'part of the *cognoscenti*[5] rather than the *illiterati*'[6] (Zappavigna 2012, p. 102, emphasis added). Despite this, internet memes lack any sense of control (Zappavigna 2012). Any offhand utterance or apparently harmless joke, once released into the networked public sphere, has the potential to endure (Van Dijck 2013). Indeed, as Perzanowski and Schultz (2016, p. 19) recently pointed out, 'it's difficult to maintain control of intellectual resources once they have been disclosed'.

Notwithstanding the enthusiasm with which the meme concept has been adopted by internet users (Shifman 2013), and the apparent connections that have been made between memes, digital culture, and learning, the field of education has been slow to catch up with the concept. A perusal of some recent books on technology in education (c.f. Ferster 2016; Garvis and Lemon 2016; Selwyn 2017, 2016; Underwood and Farrington-Flint 2015) illustrates the point, in that the term 'meme' fails to appear in most, that is, 'meme' is not in their indexes. Nevertheless, many outside formal education settings are making connections between internet memes and the ways in which young people are taking up and reshaping the way technology is used to fit their needs and expectations (boyd 2010; Jenkins *et al.* 2016, 2013; Milner 2016; Shifman 2014).

Despite the reluctance of education to connect to internet memes, young people 'simply express a need to connect' (Turkle 2011, p. 171) and the internet, alongside social media, has done much to facilitate and expedite this need. This has not happened by chance but by mutual consent (Van Dijck 2013) or at least through perceptions of autonomy. Jenkins *et al.* (2013) argue that compelling content and the need to connect combine to enhance the spreadability of cultural practice. Drawing on the work of Rushkoff (1994), Jenkins *et al.* (2013, p. 18) reason that 'the spread of ideas can often occur without the users' consent and perhaps actively against their conscious resistance'. The need to connect (Turkle 2011), the allure of social bonding (Zappavigna 2012), and the desire to be inside a social group (Shifman 2014), combine to highlight the potential power of an internet meme. There is a real risk, however, that an internet meme can 'act as a Trojan Horse', duping people into 'passing on a hidden agenda while circulating compelling content' (Jenkins *et al.* 2013, p. 17). As such, any meme has the potential to be a gift that helps young people to develop or an unwanted idea with the potential to derail their better judgement (Dennett 1991).

One of the key problems is that young people are being forced to connect and interact in the same way as adults. They are not adults, however, and should not be treated as such. Instead of applying adult rules, fears, and concepts to children and young people, we need to acknowledge that 'children overwhelmingly experience digital media as a powerful and positive influence in their daily lives' (Third *et al.* 2014, p. 12) and act accordingly.

Memes are not new. Nor are they are harmful per se. Dennett (1991) argues that human consciousness is built on cultural evolution and owes much of its progress to memes. Nevertheless, we should not assume that memes are benign, and many spread in spite of our better judgement (Dennett 1991). The proliferation and pervasiveness of the World Wide Web means that internet memes now spread in moments and are increasingly used to spread ideas that serve both for-profit businesses and government bodies. They certainly aren't designed to serve the needs of young people and it is this practice and concern that I explore in the remainder of this chapter.

Young people, social media, and internet memes

At the heart of this book are over 1,300 young people who voiced their experiences of and exposure to health-related social media. Each of these contributed – either directly or indirectly – to the six narratives, and therefore the five young people, we 'met' in Part II. Reducing the data from 1,300 individuals to five composite case studies was not easy and consequently we are left with representations of young people rather than their individual experiences. It is alongside these representations that I now seek to provide an analysis of the key findings from my perspective, through the lens of internet memes. Specifically, I will provide key interpretations of the relationship I see between the experiences of Kelly (Chapter 2) and Yaz (Chapter 3), as well as the WhatsApp discussion (Chapter 7), and my reading of the internet meme literature. I do this because I feel these three chapters best represent the types of experiences that can be scrutinised in the context of wider literature about memes and internet memes. I explore these data-rich narratives through three themes: (i) *genre of participation*, (ii) *algorithms not people as transmitters of culture*, and (iii) *adults (teachers and parents)*. In so doing, I argue for the need for new spaces in which young people and adults can explore their digital futures together.

Genre of participation

In their work about participatory culture, Jenkins *et al.* (2016, p. 60) employ the idea of 'genre of participation' to argue that young people engage in both 'interest-driven and friendship-driven participation' (p. 61) on the internet. Young people's friendship-driven participation occurs in the social networks where most of their real-life friends can be found. In contrast, their interest-driven participation is more fragmented and occurs in noticeably different online spaces and with different people focused around a common topic of interest (Jenkins *et al.* 2016).

Despite these different drivers of participation, Jenkins *et al.* (2016, pp. 63–64) identified three types of online behaviour:

> *Hanging out*: associated with friendship-driven learning and participation. It is motivated mostly by social connection and a sense of belonging.

> *Messing around*: pertaining to young people exploring and experimenting with tools and techniques as part of everyday social behaviour. Messing around is an example of how friendship-driven learning becomes a pathway to more interest-driven participation.

> *Geeking out*: encompassing young people who were driven toward gaining specialised knowledge and getting good at something. Geeking out is positioned as a springboard into interest-driven participation.

Jenkins *et al.* (2016) argued that while the same young person might engage in some or all of these genres of engagement, each young person might be dismissed by and/or experience the distain of different groups operating in other genres. It is easy to see how Kelly's (Chapter 2) uses of social media (or indeed her distain for it) could be classed as either hanging out or being seen to hang out. Indeed, the group's use of internet memes such as images and videos to communicate offers Kelly a quick and simple way of telling others that she's 'always on' even if she's not in the mood or has no Wi-Fi or data. This 'checking in' in order to 'hang out', even if she doesn't want to, forms a significant part of her online behaviour.

In contrast, Yaz's (Chapter 3) genre of engagement might have started out as 'messing around' but it has evolved into 'geeking out'. His use of the internet began as a 'search for things' but it has firmly moved to 'learning how to do stuff' in a form and through a medium that he can understand quickly and use in minutes if not seconds. Yaz's social media site of preference is YouTube rather than WhatsApp, Snapchat, or Instagram and his use is not friendship-driven but interest-driven. His friends, like Amy, get to see the results and witness his behaviour change but not the content; at least there is no indication in the narrative that Yaz is re-sharing the content he finds on YouTube and subsequently uses in the gym. Yaz is motivated to get the body he wants and is using what he can find, or what is found for him via YouTube, to transform his body.

The quality of what Yaz is sourcing however, is highly questionable. While he might be 'geeking out' he seems to be a long way away from understanding, and appropriately using the knowledge and practices he discovers. What is more, if he is re-sharing memes that are flawed, then he is guilty of passing on a hidden agenda (such as 'no pain, no gain' or, in Kelly's case, 'FitTea') without conscious resistance or relevant up-to-date knowledge.

Yaz does not judge quality by the source (i.e. a qualified fitness instructor or a government department) but by the number of likes a video receives. Worryingly, as Chapter 7 suggests, some individuals (like James) have a habit of liking everything on social media, which brings into question the trustworthiness of a measure such as likes. Indeed, Yaz's 'geeky' practices seem a long way from Jenkins *et al.*'s (2016, p. 72) aspiration that 'today's participatory culture is the site for learning to be digitally literate and net savvy, [which] can put young people on a path towards a more self-directed learning'.

Whilst Yaz and Kelly are seeing different things and in different ways, the content, form, and stance (Shifman 2014) of what they subsequently use is fairly constant. This seems almost inevitable given that algorithms appear to serve as purveyors of content rather than the specific needs or understanding of young people. Content providers may argue that they are simply playing back what young people already view, just in a different format. There is, however, a risk that individuals like Yaz and Kelly get caught in a potentially vicious circle of content with no one, outside of themselves, to regulate what they see and how they act.

Algorithms as purveyors of health and wellbeing related internet memes

There is evident conflict between young people's desire to live in and with networked publics and the desire of for-profit businesses to influence the choices that the self-same young people make. With algorithms deciding what these young people 'see' on social media is it any wonder that Kelly and Yaz are no longer required to actively search for information about health and wellbeing: it is constantly pushed at them by content providers?

Whilst we know little, if anything, about Kelly and Yaz's respective social identities we can suppose that 'what they see on their feeds, and thus what becomes normative for them, varies depending on the people in their network' (Jenkins *et al.* 2016, p. 78). Instead of helping young people like Kelly and Yaz to be self-directed learners, their exposure to parochial social feeds by social media companies does little, if anything, to realise any self-educative value of social media. In fact, it does the opposite, and goes a long way towards ensuring that these young people maintain their existing tastes and interests. Thus they become a marketer's dream, because their likes and dislikes remain unchallenged and can be easily matched to new content and new products.

The use of algorithms, coupled with young people's desires to hang out or geek out significantly reduces the meme pool – in this case for health – that was imagined by Dawkins (2006). Dawkins (1976) posited that memes would spread by leaping from brain to brain through imitation, yet it seems that social media providers are playing a disproportionately large role in determining which of the memes that Kelly and Yaz see are imitated and will therefore survive and which will not. A meme's longevity, fecundity, and copy-fidelity is no longer determined by chance. It does not come down to the compelling nature of the content either. Increasingly, it would seem, it comes down to the types of users in any given network and the ways in which for-profit businesses can leverage them. Consequently, cultural evolution increasingly comes with £ and $ signs attached.

Shifman (2014, p. 71) showed that 'approaching the right people is critical in the viral process' especially at a time when for-profit businesses are seeking ways of determining any given meme's success. Seeding ideas that can jump from brain to brain can be facilitated by hubs; that is, 'people with high numbers of connections to others' and bridges; that is, 'people who connect between otherwise unconnected parts of the network' (ibid., p. 71). The use of such hubs and bridges, however, gives little, if any, consideration to the occupants of such networks, the manner in which networks overlap and intertwine, and the vulnerability of any young people involved in these networks. In short, an 'age-generic (or "age-blind") approach to [network] users' appears to have been taken in these cases' (Livingstone *et al.* 2016, p. 1). Put differently, businesses are concerned with reaching the masses as quickly as possible and give little thought to individuals.

Memes have been studied because they reflect contemporary cultural, social, and political practice (Shifman 2014). Perhaps internet memes should be studied because they are being commandeered for economic gain. If, as Dawkins (2006, p. 46) suggested, 'the gene is the basic unit of selfishness' then perhaps the internet meme is too. Indeed, whilst Milner (2016, p. 2) argued that 'when everyday members of the public contribute their small conversational strands to the vast tapestry, they are memetically making their world', the greater concern is how much freedom individuals still have in making their individual contributions.

It is unlikely that any of the young people in this book are either hubs or bridges, but the presence of either or both in their respective networks will impact on the memetic content they see. That is not to say that Kelly or Yaz or indeed any of the individuals in the WhatsApp conversation (Chapter 7) have no impact on their social networks, but the presence of commercial interests, via celebrity or branding, certainly skews what they might see. While we should not assume that young people are savvy to the nuances of internet memes, nor should we assume they are not. Equally we should not assume that all young people benefit from the input of adults, nor that adults are always ignorant of what happens on social media.

Adults: teachers and parents

Traditionally, adults have been perceived to 'know best' because they simply have more life experience and understand the dangers of the world better. Such behaviour is seen both in the research around networked participation and internet memes and in the WhatsApp group in Chapter 7.

A key finding from Chapter 7 was that parent/ guardians and schools/ teachers are ill-equipped to support young people to make informed decisions about the health-related material they access and attend to on social media. In some ways, this finding is a memetic construction and in other ways it reflects the dearth of cultural understanding that adults have about the world in which young people live.

When the WhatsApp group brands the school's attempts to educate them about participating in social media as 'irrelevant' they reflect the memetic idea that adults are irrelevant and under-informed. Which generation has ever seen their schools, teachers, parents, or guardians as relevant or understanding of popular culture? It is improbable that the friendship-driven participation of the young people in this book, via mechanisms such as hanging out and messing around (Jenkins *et al.* 2016), would see them defending the adults in their lives, even if they wanted to. Such a move would be paramount to social suicide.

The flipside to the above argument seems to be the assumptions that adults make about social media. Many have argued that the internet and social media have been overly positioned as sinister (see: Livingstone, Carr, and Byrne 2016, Swift and Collin 2017, Third *et al.* 2014). The dark side of the web popularises – indeed makes a meme of – the idea that young people are at new and enduring risk because they are 'always on' social media (boyd 2014, p. 211). There is a memetic expectation that young people are more readily exposed to violence and inappropriate content, goods and services, they are prone to technology over-use, and they have poor data protection and privacy practices (Third *et al.* 2014).

The combination of heightened opportunity and poor practice – or at least adults' expectations of it – seem to be responsible for the latest in a series of 'running joke' assemblies about internet safety reported in Chapter 7. In this chapter, the school's assumption seemed to be that one person's bad experience is representative of everyone else's experiences. It is this assumption that prompts teachers to reemphasise old messages about privacy settings and cyber-bullying, rather than dealing with real issues such as peer pressure and all the images of perfect bodies with which the WhatsApp group are bombarded.

Whilst both adults and young people are caught in a memetic cliché, it is clear that the teachers should have responded differently. Whilst parents and guardians may have been placated because the school had immediately called an assembly and reiterated the messages about safety, this has previously been proven to have little impact. In the same way that young people expect adults not to understand, so adults expect, and are expected, to assume that young people are guilty of poor practice and, therefore, at fault.

Implications for addressing young people, social media, and internet memes

Memes and internet memes

Many of the concerns highlighted in this book are in and of themselves memes and 'reflect deep social and cultural structures' (Shifman 2014, p. 15). The very name of the WhatsApp group in Chapter 7 serves to highlight the gulf of expectation and understanding between adults and young people (i.e. Kelly, Yaz, Leah, James, and Jess). Furthermore, the age-related disparagement of the young by the old, and vice versa, is another deep cultural structure. It is no easy undertaking to shift expectations about knowledge and understanding; but shifted they must be.

If internet memes are being created to deliberately carry political, corporate, economic, or other agendas and priorities and are not tailored to or created by young people, then they have the potential to do harm on a large scale. While internet memes have been positioned as 'meaningless media snacks' (Shifman 2014, p. 11) the increasing desire of marketers to 'make memes go viral' (Jenkins, Ford, and Green 2013, p. 5) so big business can influence the decisions of young people changes the landscape. That said, it is not enough to assume ignorance on the part of young people, nor is it enough for adults to roll out the expected response and hope for different results. Things need to change on both sides of the equation.

From my perspective as a teacher-educator motivated to help young people, and as a father playing a role in the development of two young people in a digital landscape, I am concerned at the potential of social media to place young people at risk. I am keen to play a part in 're-scripting digital education as a site for sustained public debate and political controversy' (Selwyn 2016, p. 149). When we employ an 'age blind' approach to internet governance (Livingstone, Carr, and Byrne 2016, p. 1) and fail to include young people's voices in our debates, we also fail to 'learn to understand digital media through children's eyes' (Swift and Collin 2017, p. 12). We must be mindful that young people engage in social media, and *ergo* interact with internet memes, in different ways and for different purposes. They are not an homogeneous group who need a blanket response, but are individuals with bespoke needs.

Genre of engagement

Young people are not passive users of social media. Instead they engage in complex social processes that define their world and encapsulate their experiences. It is hard to imagine a major cultural or political event that does not inspire its own memes. Consequently, it is vital that, as adults, we better understand how young people seek to raise their 'cool quotient' (Zappavigna 2012, p. 101) and be cognisant of the diverse ways in which they 'hang out', 'mess around' and 'geek out' (Jenkins *et al.* 2016, pp. 63–64) while trying to stay safe. Based on the findings reported in the case study chapters (Chapters 2–7), young people actively seek to place themselves in dangerous situations on social media. Consequently, we must be mindful that activity on social media doesn't simply equate to danger. If we don't share, and don't seek to understand, each other's cultural practices then we are doomed to remain caught in the memes of our own making; that is, the belief that neither party understands or 'gets' the other.

Young people should be seen and should be heard and the solution to any act of folly, or indeed misfortune as in the case of the anorexia sufferer (Chapter 5), should not be to assume the worst and remove the potential for further engagement in these communities. Given the social significance of simply checking in to tell people why you can't be on Snapchat or Instagram – which in itself seems like an oxymoron – what are the consequences of untethering a young person from that network? Jenkins *et al.* (2016) argued that some of the most innovative uses of the internet and digital technology occur when young people seek to circumnavigate firewalls and other preventive measures imposed on them by adults. What is to stop young people taking greater risks to overcome adult-imposed obstacles? If we take away access to social media, we are backing young people into a corner and challenging them to find innovative ways of checking in anyway. It lies with us as adults to find ways of understanding young people's needs and managing our expectations accordingly, rather than instigating a blanket ban that could have huge impact on young people's carefully managed social networks.

Algorithms as purveyors of health and wellbeing related internet memes

According to Kelly (Chapter 2) we are 'mad' to consider a world where social media does not play a significant part in the lives of young people. Algorithms seem to be the very antithesis of education and yet they seem to be key in deciding what sources of health and wellbeing knowledge young people are seeing. Whilst 'in the Dawkinism sense, meme labels units of cultural transmission, but its application to what we call internet memes raises critical questions about individual agency in the spread of information' (Milner 2016, p. 15, original emphasis). In this context, it would seem that internet memes are not so much 'cultural touchstones' (Milner 2016) as they are entrepreneurial steers and, as adults, we need to be aware of this.

Adults: teachers and parents

In their work exploring young people and their engagement with health-related social media, Goodyear, Armour, and Wood (2018, p. 15) concluded that:

> Given the challenges that many relevant adults face in understanding social media, young people currently lack appropriate guidance in their health-related uses of social media. In particular, young people need the kind of support that is responsive to those points in time when young people tip from being in control of the media, to the media controlling them.

In considering the spaces in which young people now operate it is no longer acceptable for adults to be either outsiders or intruders in the digital lives of young people. As Kelly argued in Chapter 7, young people need to tell adults about the 'problems of our generation' and help adults to be 'made aware of the risks' young people face so that they can 'check if we are struggling'. That does not mean that adults should follow memetic protocol and disconnect young people from their networks. Rather than seeking to exclude young people from the decision-making process adults must, instead, endeavour to support young people as they negotiate these spaces.

Turkle (2011, p. 173) has argued that technology has muddled the 'rite of passage' from childhood to adulthood. Where, a generation ago, children would eventually be set free to travel alone – albeit to the local town centre – now they are habitually tethered to their parent through the mobile phones they carry but for which their parent or guardian pays. The parental contract that comes with this financial and connective benefit is often the expectation of parents or guardians that they are brought along as their children explore increasing distant spaces (Turkle 2011). In short, there seems to an ongoing parental need to protect young people from stranger-danger, the dark side of the web, and the like. However, this seems to equate to fear of a space – a digital space in this case – that parents and teachers do not occupy, do not understand, cannot navigate, and where anything they profess to know is deemed as irrelevant and outdated by those they are seeking to protect.

The findings represented in the six case study narratives (Chapters 2–7) suggest the need for new forms of, and forums for, adult education. Such sites would help adults challenge their status as tourist, acknowledge their inadequacies and ignorance (at least from the perceptions of young people), and help them to understand the world in which young people live. Such openness could work both ways, and help young and older alike to see the memetic constructions of age that stop them conversing in meaningful ways. Finally, it would help both groups to collectively challenge the role social media marketers and algorithm writers play in spreading messages about health and wellbeing.

Summary of key messages

- Memes and internet – Memes are key structures in cultural transmission. Whilst not new – Dawkins (1976) would argue that they have been around for millennia – their spread (i.e. their longevity, fecundity, and copy-fidelity) is being expedited by the vast social networks that exist on the internet. The spread of a meme is now measured in minutes and hours rather than days and weeks, and it is important that young people and adults alike are mindful of the speed of transmission. Equally, given the accelerated nature of meme replication, there is less time for meme recipients to gauge the 'quality' of what they are seeing. This, in turn, places young people at greater risk of sharing a potential 'Trojan Horse' and, in so doing, 'pass on a hidden agenda while circulating compelling content' (Jenkins *et al.* 2013, p. 17).

- Genre of participation – Young people use social media for different reasons and in different ways. It is not enough to opt for a homogenous approach to young people's uses of such platforms. As adults, we must be aware that young people either already 'get it' (i.e. the inside joke) or they desire to be 'part of it' and show they are 'like you [those on the inside]' (Zappavigna 2012). Additionally, we need to be aware of different friendship-driven and interest-driven networked publics and be mindful of how they may influence what young people are experiencing/seeing on the internet.

- Algorithms not people as transmitters of culture – Increasingly, it seems, young people are not as involved as they might wish to be in choosing what they and their friends see on social media. Content is being chosen and manufactured by others. Despite young people's belief that 'likes' are a suitable yardstick of quality; social media companies and big businesses are finding ways of circumnavigating or influencing the cultural messages young people see and potentially interact with. The spread from network to network is algorithmically enhanced and is not a true reflection of what young people understand and believe. It is important that we do not take young people's feeds at face-value because, in doing so, we run a very real risk of homogenising them rather than seeing and comprehending their individuality.

- Adults: teachers and parents – Understanding the memes that surround young and older people alike allows us to comprehend our own prejudices and predispositions. Then, in comprehending our biases, we can begin to overcome them. The young people represented in the first part of this book are seen to be frustrated by what they see as poor understanding of social media. They are irritated that adults' responses to perceived danger are irrelevant and outdated, whilst simultaneously wishing adults would increase their awareness of how young people use social media, the risks they face, and the ways they might navigate these risks. New spaces are needed for these difficult conversations, spaces that acknowledge and seek to overcome existing cultural memes about age, wisdom, and danger, and allow both parties to explore new futures where the voices of young people are central to any discussions and actions pertaining to social media.

Notes

1 https://en.wikipedia.org/wiki/Ice_Bucket_Challenge
2 https://en.wikipedia.org/wiki/Success_Kid
3 Networked publics are publics that are restructured by networked technologies ... they allow people to gather for social, cultural, and civic purposes and they help people connect with a world beyond their close friends and family (boyd 2010, p. 39).
4 A language that is adopted as a common language between speakers whose native languages are different (Oxford Living Dictionaries 2018).
5 People who are especially well informed about a particular subject.
6 People who are not well educated or well informed about a particular subject or sphere of activity.

References

Blackmore, S., 1999. *The Meme Machine*. Oxford, UK: Oxford University Press.

boyd, d., 2010. Social network sites as networked publics: affordances, dynamics, and Implications. *In:* Zizi Papacharissi, ed., *Networked Self: Identity, Community, and Culture on Social Network Sites*, pp. 39–58 (accessed 1 November 2017 www.danah.org/papers/2010/SNSasNetworkedPublics.pdf).

boyd, d., 2014. *It's Complicated: The Social Lives of Networked Teens*. New Haven, CT: Yale University Press.

Dawkins, R., 1976. *The Selfish Gene*. Oxford, UK: Oxford University Press.

Dawkins, R., 2006. *The Selfish Gene*. Oxford, UK: Oxford University Press.

Dennett, D.C., 2017. *From Bacteria to Bach and Back: The Evolution of Minds*. London: Penguin Books.

Dennett, D.C., 1991. *Consciousness Explained*. London: Penguin Books.

Ferster, B., 2016. *The Sage on the Screen: Education, Media, and How to Learn.* Baltimore, MD: Johns Hopkins University Press.

Garvis, S. and Lemon, N., 2016. *Understanding Digital Technologies and Young Children: An International Perspective.* London, UK: Routledge.

Godwin, M., 1994. Meme, Counter-meme. *Wired* (accessed 25 January 2018 www.wired.com/wired/archive/2.10/godwin.if.html).

Goodyear, V.A., Armour, K.M., and Wood, H., 2018. Young people and their engagement with health-related social media: New perspectives. *Sport, Education and Society*, iFirst Article.

Jenkins, H., Ito, M., and boyd, d., 2016. *Participatory Culture in Networked Era: A Conversation on Youth, Learning, Commerce and Politics*. Cambridge: Polity Press.

Jenkins, H., Ford, S., and Green, J., 2013. *Spreadable Media: Creating Value and Meaning in Networked Culture.* New York: New York University Press.

Kirk, D., 2010. *Physical Education Futures*. London, UK: Routledge.

Livingstone, S., Carr, J., and Byrne, J., 2016. One in three: Internet governance and children's rights. *Innocenti Discussion Paper* No. 2016–01, UNICEF Office of Research, Florence.

Lynch, A., 1996. *Thought Contagion: How Belief Spreads Through Society*. New York, NY: Basic Books.

Milner, R.M., 2016. *The World Made Meme: Public Conversations and Participatory Media.* Cambridge, MA: MIT Press.

Nahon, K. and Hemsley, J., 2013. *Going Viral*. Cambridge, UK: Polity Press.

Perzanowski, A. and Schultz, J.M., 2016. *The End of Ownership: Personal Property in the Digital Economy*. Cambridge, MA: MIT Press.

Selwyn, N., 2017. *Education and Technology: Key Issues and Debates*. London, UK: Bloomsbury.

Selwyn, N., 2016. *Is Technology Good for Education?* Cambridge, UK: Polity Press.

Shifman, L., 2014. *Memes in Digital Culture*. Cambridge, MA: MIT Press.

Shifman, L., 2013. Memes in a digital world: reconciling with a conceptual troublemaker. *Journal of Computer-Mediated Communication*, 18, 362–377.

Solon, O., 2013. Richard Dawkins on the internet's hijacking of the word 'meme'. *Wired* (accessed 25 January 2018 www.wired.co.uk/article/richard-dawkins-memes).

Swift, T. and Collin, P., 2017. Platforms, data and children's rights: Introducing a 'networked capability approach'. *New Media & Society*, 19(5), 671–685.

Third, A., Bellerose, D., Dawkins, U., Keltie, E., and Pihl, K., 2014. *Children's Rights in the Digital Age: A Download from Children Around the World*. Melbourne: Young and Well Cooperative Research Centre.

Tinning, R., 2014. The obesity crisis and the field of kinesiology: A discursive and memetic consideration. *Quest*, 66(1), 27–38.

Tinning, R., 2012. The idea of physical education: A memetic perspective. *Physical Education and Sport Pedagogy*, 17(2), 115–126.

Turkle, S., 2011. *Alone Together: Why We Expect More Technology and Less From Each Other*. New York: Basic Books.

Tuten, T. and Solomon, M., 2012. *Social Media Marketing*. Englewood Cliffs, NJ: Prentice Hall.

Underwood, J.D.M. and Farrington-Flint, L., 2015. *Learning and the E-Generation*. Oxford, UK: Wiley Blackwell.

Van Dijck, J., 2013. *The Culture of Connectivity: A Critical History of Social Media*. Oxford, UK: Oxford University Press.

Zappavigna, M., 2012. *Discourse of Twitter and Social Media: How We use Language to Create Affiliation on the Web*. London, UK: Bloomsbury.

15 Young people, social media, and digital democracy

Towards a participatory foundation for health and physical education's engagement with digital technologies

Eimear Enright and Michael Gard

Chapter overview

In this chapter we seek to offer new pedagogical pathways for a student-driven, digital health and physical education (HPE). We do this by bringing the democratic affordances of digital technologies into dialogue with the democratic impulse of education and by proposing a democratic and participatory foundation for HPE's engagement with digital technologies.

Digital democracy

Last year, we went to see the Irish comedian David O'Doherty perform in a Brisbane theatre. Taking to the stage with his signature half-sized, electronic keyboard, O'Doherty engaged us in an irreverent reflection on the trials and tribulations of modern life. A highlight for us, and for the audience judging from the reaction, was O'Doherty's perspective on the internet. He argued that the internet had morphed from an amazing telescope through which we might learn about all the incredible possibilities that the universe has to offer, into an enormous 'shitpipe' that pumps a constant flow of excrement at us, and even though we don't like it, we are all so addicted we now have no choice but to submit. Through laughter-induced tears, one of our dear friends turned to us and said, 'so true'.

You might wonder why this scene from our social lives is relevant to you, or to this chapter. It is relevant because the seasoned comedian so easily constructed both the internet and its users in negative and deficit ways, and because these constructions had mass appeal. But, these constructions, although humorous, were incomplete. In this chapter we want to tell a more balanced story of the affordances of digital technologies[1] and present a more nuanced and agentic construction of its users. By bringing the democratic affordances of digital technologies into dialogue with the democratic impulse of education, we also seek to offer new pedagogical pathways for a student-driven, digital health and physical education (HPE).[2]

There is a sustained and growing body of scholarship that suggests developments in digital technology signal the potential for 'quantum leaps in the field of democratic politics' (Becker 1998, p. 343), as opportunities hitherto unavailable to rethink, overhaul, or replace anti-democratic actors, practices, and institutions become available (Hague and Loader 1999, Kahne, Middaugh, and Allen 2015). While numerous initiatives and models have emerged that try to advocate for and/or describe this reinvigoration of democratic practices through digital technologies (e.g. teledemocracy, cyberdemocracy, e-democracy), we prefer the term digital democracy as it encompasses a broader range of technological applications (Hague and Loader 1999). This term is, however, necessarily nebulous, because assumptions about democracy and democratic subjectivity will always affect how an individual constructs the democratic affordances of digital tools (Dahlberg 2011). That being said, for the purposes of this chapter, we understand digital democracy as inclusive of all of the ways in which digital technologies might be used to promote democratic values (such as justice, equality, autonomy, freedom), enhance governance processes, and support greater participation by all citizens in accessing knowledge, debating, expressing opinions, and making meaningful contributions to the decisions that shape their lives (Dahlberg 2011; Hague and Loader 1999; Montgomery 2008).

We are neither technology evangelists nor naïve techno-optimists. We do not extol the potential of digital technologies because we believe that recruiting digital technologies will simply transfer the balance of power to the demos. Indeed, like many others, we are aware and sceptical of the grandiose assertions and hyperbolic claims being made about digital democracy (Hague and Loader 1999) and the emancipatory potential of the internet and other 'liberation technologies' (Diamond 2010, p. 69). We are sceptical because we know, for example, that many young people are systematically denied access to digital technologies on the basis of economic status, gender, geographic location, and so on (Liao *et al.* 2016), that even the most open protocols and the cheapest hardware do not eliminate equalities associated with creating or accessing particular content (Hindman 2008), that many anti-democratic and harmful offline behaviours (e.g. 'traditional' bullying) are now finding an equally, if not more damaging online expression (e.g. cyberbullying) (Waasdorp and Bradshaw 2015), and that invisible personalisation biases what we access and limits opportunities for the democratic exchange of ideas on every major website (Pariser 2011). We also know that to some degree, O'Doherty's construction of the internet as a 'shitpipe' holds true, as one function of the internet seems to be to 'pump' junk or spam at us (Ferrara 2017). Moreover, work across many diverse contexts (e.g. military technology, climate change) and the recent data harvesting scandal,[3] has taught us that technology may ultimately prove unreliable in the pursuit of a more just and democratic world (Bernstein 2004; Stern 2007; Summers 2018).

That being said, we still see digital technologies as tools capable of being shaped in the pursuit of more democratic goals and pedagogies. Our reasons for this are multiple but coalesce around the high and sustained use of digital technologies by young people (Australian Bureau of Statistics (ABS) 2017; Third *et al.* 2017), and the open and collaborative networking characteristics of many digital technologies (Loader and Mercea 2011). In Australia (where we live) and internationally, young people aged 15 to 24 are reported to access the internet more than any other age group (International Telecommunications Union 2013). Recent statistics highlight that in 2014–2015, while 85 per cent of persons in Australia were internet users, the 15–17 year age group had the highest proportion of internet use (at 99%). This age group also spent the highest number of hours per week (18 hours) on the internet (ABS 2017). In recent years, there has also been a significant change in how young people access the internet. They are now more likely to access the internet via a smartphone than through personal computers or laptops, and they often have multiple access options. The 2014–2015 data reveals that for households with children aged under 15 years, the mean number of devices used to access the internet at home was seven (ABS 2017). Thus, while we are conscious that there are young people in the minority and majority world who do not have easy and ongoing access to digital technologies, for many young people a plethora of digital tools and contexts for accessing, discussing, and producing information are available, and are being used anonymously and on demand.

Research on young people's engagement across various digital mediascapes identifies a number of core interactive and dialogic practices (Kahn, Middaugh, and Allen 2015). Many young people, for example, readily recruit digital technologies, individually and in groups, to pursue their interests, to circulate information, to socialise, collaborate, create, debate, advocate, and to learn (Bessant 2014; Kahn, Middaugh, and Allen 2015). These kinds of cultural practices create spaces that are filled with new possibilities to deepen, expand, and in some cases revive democracy (Bessant 2014). That is not to say that this is, or can ever be, a guaranteed or straightforward process.

Digital technologies, whether directed at enhancing democracy or not, 'emerge out of the dialectical interaction between technology and society' (Castells 1997, p. 5), and 'will be shaped through the activities of human agents, constrained as they are by existing power relations' (Hague and Loader 1999, p. 4). We have written elsewhere about the increasing interest in the use of digital technologies and we have shared our concerns that the transformative and democratic potential of digital technologies might be squandered (Enright *et al.* 2016). This is also a conversation worth revisiting and extending in this chapter. Recognising how and by whom the construction and use of digital technologies in schools (and in HPE specifically) is shaped is an important context for a chapter that engages with the concept of democracy and proposes how things might be theorised and practiced differently.

On the one hand, Gard (2014) has described some of the ways in which digital technologies are currently being used in an essentially punitive manner to make schools and students more accountable for public health outcomes. On the other hand, there is the less dramatic but equally unfortunate possibility that digital technologies will be used in HPE to deliver more of the same (Enright *et al.* 2016), an outcome that has regularly been described in other curriculum areas by educational researchers (Selwyn 2010; Smeets 2005). Indeed, the gulf between the transformative promises and claims made for the use of digital technologies in schools, and the translation of these into actual classroom practices remains significant (Sanders and George 2017; Selwyn 2010).

There are many factors that have pushed, and appear likely to continue to push, the use of digital technologies in HPE in an educationally conservative direction. For example, the influence of public health agendas, while well meaning, have encouraged some researchers and teachers to see digital technology merely as a tool for 'fixing' young people (Vander Shee and Boyles 2010). In particular, mobile applications (apps) and devices that require teachers and students to record a huge range of health and physical activity-related data are proliferating (Lupton 2013; Rich and Miah 2017). While these apps and devices may have their place in the lives of people who have decided to monitor or change their lifestyle, their educational value is less clear (Gard and Enright 2016).

It is also worth keeping in mind that schools across the Western world are increasingly being seen by businesses as markets to be exploited, and this perhaps is nowhere more apparent than in the commerce of digital technology (Enright *et al.* 2016; Gard 2014; Vander Shee and Boyles 2010). In fact, the fusing of private enterprise with public health agendas – such as those focused on obesity and mental health – is now being exploited by a wide range of commercially motivated educational resource providers (Enright *et al.* 2016; Fullagar *et al.* 2017). Digital technology is at the heart of these enterprises.

Meanwhile, the question of HPE's relevance to young people remains a pressing concern for the field (Enright and O'Sullivan 2012; Gard, Hickey-Moody, and Enright 2013). Perhaps at its most fundamental, this tension arises when a curriculum area is heavily influenced by a top-down agenda, such as that embodied by public health, that makes a priori assumptions about what young people need and what they should know. Taking HPE fields like drug and alcohol education and sexuality education, however, it is clear that these assumptions can be inaccurate and even misguided, and are often grounded in a deficit view of young people and their health (Leahy *et al.* 2015). Not surprisingly then, some of the growing interest in using digital technology in HPE also reflects this top-down/deficit starting point. In other words, many advocates for the use of digital technologies in HPE simply see it as a vehicle for intensifying a long-standing and yet perennially unfulfilled mission to 'save' young people (Gard and Pluim 2014).

Outside of HPE, studies have historically found that parents (Ackard and Neumark-Sztainer 2001) and peers (Gould and Mazzeo 1982) have been young people's primary sources of health information. Since the early 2000s however, research on young people's health information-seeking behaviours has highlighted that digital media, including the internet (Gray *et al.* 2005; Third *et al.* 2017) and mobile applications (e.g. Gard and Enright 2016), are increasingly significant spaces for young people to seek out information on a variety of health-related topics (Swist *et al.* 2015).

There is now a growing body of literature that seeks to map and analyse young people's access to, and engagement with, digital tools and contexts for health-related purposes (Burns *et al.* 2010; Swist *et al.* 2015; Wartella *et al.* 2016). However, the vast majority of studies into young people's access to online health information, particularly sexual and mental health information, have focused on the apparent 'quality' or 'credibility' (or lack thereof) of information (Eysenbach 2008; Freeman *et al.* 2018). The recommendations from these studies are usually couched in risk discourses and generally advocate for an improvement in the 'accuracy' or quality of online health information (Hausmann *et al.* 2017; Mitchell *et al.* 2014), better tailored health information to reflect young people's concerns and interests (Beck *et al.* 2014), and interventions that improve the 'digital literacy'[4] (St. Jean *et al.* 2015) or 'eHealth literacy'[5] (Freeman *et al.* 2018; Neter and Brainin 2012) of young people. Each of these popular recommendations are problematic; first because it is neither possible nor desirable to censor all young people's access to digital health networks; second because it assumes a generic young person that online health information can be targeted at; and third because it is grounded in a belief that young people have significant deficiencies regarding health literacy skills and/or digital literacy skills and that they are only capable of naïve readings of digital health media. We should highlight here that the tide has begun to turn. There are an increasing number of articles and reports that now also acknowledge digital technologies, and in particular social media, as a health resource and recognise positive ways in which young people use and benefit from them (e.g. Frith 2017; Goodyear, Armour, and Wood 2018). However, risk and deficit discourses do still dominate in the vast majority of studies that have young people's health-related behaviours as a focus.

In contrast, there is a large and vibrant research literature concerned with exploring youth voice, digital technologies, and digital culture more broadly, that tends to be more nuanced in its treatment of young people's engagement with technology. Indeed, an increasing number of scholars, across a host of disciplines (e.g. education, media studies, youth studies, politics, sociology, physical education and sport pedagogy, leisure studies) recognise that as active constructors of digital culture, young people are increasingly blogging, vlogging, tweeting, developing their own websites, and creating new kinds of digital media subcultures (Buckingham and Willet 2013; Kenway and Bullen 2008; Enright and Gard 2015; Sefton-Green 2004; Montgomery 2008). These scholars acknowledge that many young people have grown up in a media landscape that has been digitally transformed, and are realising the participatory, democratic, and transformative capabilities of digital media (Buckingham 2008; Montgomery 2008; Selwyn 2010). Therefore, rather than taking risk, crisis, or concern (Beck 1992) as a starting point, or allowing risk-related discourses to dominate, these scholars often begin with a recognition of young people as active social agents, critical observers, and cultural producers (Buckingham and Willet 2013; Kenway and Bullen 2008; Sefton-Green 2004). This is very much a strengths-based orientation to young people's engagement with digital culture. Unsurprisingly, this scholarship is also far more likely to acknowledge the democratising potential of the internet and advocate for critical, post critical (Kenway and Bullen 2008), dialogical, and participatory pedagogies (Asthana 2009; Roberts-Holmes 2014), as opposed to draconian censorship.

The background to this chapter, then, is a mixture of challenges and opportunities. Yes, there are dangers and risks associated with young people's online engagement, and these have been well documented and should not be ignored. However, digital technologies can be tools for democratic enhancement (Buckingham 2015; Loader and Mercea 2011), if they afford the opportunity for young people to access information, express opinions, debate, participate in governance, create and challenge content, and be heard and responded to in decision-making. While there are obvious dangers in constructing it as an educational panacea, the ubiquity, flexibility, and utility of digital technology suggest a wide range of unrealised democratic and pedagogical possibilities that begin with the wisdom young people have about their bodies, and resonate with their digital experiences and practices.

Young people, social media, and digital democracy

We approached the case study chapters (Chapters 2–7) with an appreciation of the contours of a number of the debates about young people, health, and technology. We recruited the idea of digital democracy as our theoretical touchstone and were unapologetically looking for examples in the cases of young people exploiting the participatory capabilities of digital media (Montgomery 2008). We were seeking a sense of critical agency in the data, expecting, perhaps, to read about young citizen-users not only being offered, but also creating new opportunities for challenging dominant discourses and privileged positions of power and engaging in lifestyle and identity politics (Dahlgren 2009, Loader and Mercea 2011). Given the size of the data set (>1,300 young people) and our reading and previous research (Enright and Gard 2015), we thought we might access compelling evidence that at least some young people were expressing and creating alternative perspectives and using multimedia formats (e.g. audio and video, image and text etc.) and postmodern design methods (e.g. bricolage, parody) to articulate critique (Kenway and Bullen 2008). We were asked by the editors to pay particular attention to Chapters 2, 4, and 7.

From the first line of the first case (Kelly, Chapter 2) it became clear to us that in some ways we would be traversing old ground. The opening sentence to Chapter 2 alerts us that the chapter will engage with 'the finding that young people are open and vulnerable to rampant commercialism on social media'. What follows is a narrative that, sadly, does little to convince the reader of Kelly's developed critical facility, nor of her sense of agency. If one was looking for compelling evidence of subversion, politicisation, or contestation of dominant and harmful ideologies and practices, they would not find it in Kelly's narrative.

To be clear, we do not question the analytical approach that resulted in this narrative. The authors undertook a rigorous analysis of their data (Goodyear, Armour, and Wood 2018) and have constructed credible characters. Neither, are we suggesting that Kelly is a totally naïve consumer of the images and videos related to health that she engages with. Kelly does have some critical distance from the social media she consumes. She says, for example, that some of the content 'sends the wrong message and makes it look as if there are shortcuts to a healthy life'. She also chooses to ignore posts about health, and this strategy could easily be construed as an act of resistance. We were, however, disappointed (as perhaps the researchers who led this project were here) not to access more compelling evidence of young people harnessing digital technologies in ways that significantly enhanced insight and learning about their health, their bodies, and their worlds.

The stakeholder responses to Kelly's narrative (Chapter 2), which open with an acknowledgement of the potentially positive impact of social media on peer relationships, very quickly reveal key concerns about the 'risk-related' impacts on youth, and construct youth as 'naïve' and as 'easy commercial targets'. Moreover, one of the main considerations arrived at is that 'young people and adults need to be better informed about the risk-related impacts of social media on young people's health and wellbeing'. Given Kelly's narrative, and our prior engagement with a selection of literature on young people, technology, and health (e.g. Beck *et al.* 2014; Eysenbach 2008; Freeman *et al.* 2018; Mitchell *et al.* 2014; Neter and Brainin 2012), where deficit constructions of youth dominated, we were not surprised by this analysis, nor by the recommendations arrived at. It is one story of the data.

In Chapter 4, the character of Leah is used to communicate how social media intensifies the opportunities for peer comparison. The introduction to the chapter acknowledges young people as cultural producers, but very quickly frames this production in negative terms, linking it to heightened levels of body dissatisfaction. Similar to Kelly (Chapter 2), Leah's character emerges as more of a follower, than a subversive, and similar to Kelly's narrative, the negative consequences drive the story. Again, while we might be disappointed with the way in which the narrative was framed, body dissatisfaction was clearly a strong theme constructed through analysis. There was some evidence of criticality in Leah's narrative. For example, she explicitly constructed the images she saw on social media as a form of peer pressure. Leah and Chloe's Snapchat dialogue also revealed how peer interaction on social media can enhance empathy and support diversity. So, while there may not have been much evidence of participants scripting themselves differently by, for example, hijacking social media and actively curating digital culture (Enright 2013) to transgress and disrupt harmful gendered stereotypes (Buckingham and Willet 2013; Kenway and Bullen 2008; Sefton-Green 2004), small, potentially powerful acts of disruption did shine through in Leah's narrative.

We turn now to the stakeholder response in Chapter 4. Again, similar to that shared in Chapter 2, this response was couched in risk discourses. This time the focus was the negative consequences of social comparison and, specifically, 'peer-to-peer body comparison' as a 'risky behaviour that stems from young people's uses of social media'. We are also told in Chapter 4 that young people need to develop resilience and empathy and 'be supported to celebrate diversity and not reject it'. While it is necessary to highlight that the stakeholders were supportive of young people's uses of social media and saw it as an opportunity for health, the stakeholders' responses, across both of our reviewed chapters, were more focused on young people's vulnerability, and less on their agency. The reference to Chloe's resilience (in dialogue with Leah, Chapter 4) aside, there was limited support in the stakeholder responses for the idea that all young people have particular strengths, interests, resources, and competencies that they can and do draw on to enhance their own and others' health and wellbeing. We are not saying that the narratives or the responses were all doom and gloom. Reading outside of our assigned narratives revealed that young people in the data set were, for example, 'tactically manipulating the functions of social media' (James' friends, Chapter 5) and engaging with social media to help them learn (Yaz, Chapter 3). There was, therefore, some evidence of both critical analysis and creative production, but this tended to be muted.

Chapter 7, in some ways, speaks back to this critique and turns the tables on the stakeholders' responses. The first key finding shared here is that young people believe that adults over-estimate the risks of social media due to a lack of understanding. This is significant for two reasons. First, because the young people are asking for a certain degree of moderation in terms of the risk discourses adults draw on and reproduce. Second, because here we see the young people construct adults in deficit terms. Also significant in Chapter 7 is that while there is clearly a lack of certainty about how to address the problems that have been constructed, there is the suggestion that a different kind of health education might be necessary in schools.

Indeed, for us, what the narratives and responses provoked were questions about what kind of HPE might contribute to the construction of more positive stories about young people who are actively celebrating, enjoying, and utilising social media to blend politics with pleasure, who are more astute in their critique of the connections between production and consumption, and who are intellectually curious, active, and ethical citizens. We believe one possible answer to this question is an HPE that is biased towards rich, inclusive, democratic, and non-deficit educational experiences. To co-create this kind of HPE, we propose that we need different starting points for our research and our pedagogies. A more focused and sensitised early emphasis on, and engagement with, what students and teachers appreciate about their experiences of using digital technologies for health could facilitate a co-constructive process of theory building that attempts to build on, rather than repair, what is (Enright *et al.* 2014), and assist students, teachers, and researchers in working together to flesh out stories of success. These stories, like their deficit counterparts, will still only offer a partial account of the subject matter, but they may serve to disrupt dominant narratives, and offer new contexts and opportunities for educative work.

Implications for addressing young people, social media, and digital democracy

Mobilising students' voices in pedagogical innovation

Arguably, what is missing from the multiple rationales and arguments crafted for the use of digital technologies in HPE is an educationally democratic impulse. We strongly believe that students need to be located at the heart of much needed HPE pedagogical innovation and that we, the physical education and sport pedagogy research community, need to map and learn from the *process* of these kinds of pedagogical innovations. We need to build new knowledge about the constraints, risks, and possibilities for student-led innovation in HPE (Coll *et al.* 2018; Enright and O'Sullivan 2010a, 2010b, 2012). We currently know very little about the ways in which students would *prefer* to use digital technologies in HPE. This is not to suggest that student preference should be the overriding consideration in pedagogical innovation. At the same time, it is increasingly apparent that HPE faces an 'old wine in new bottles' problem in which digital technologies are overwhelmingly being used to transfer existing pedagogical assumptions from one medium (for example, paper) to another (computer screens) (Gard 2014). Food education is a powerful example of this. Apps and online games have proliferated which simply replicate the pen-and-paper activities of the past that asked students to count the calories they consume and develop hypothetical meals based on 'correct' choices about food types and proportions (Gard and Enright 2016). Apart from their simplistic didacticism, these approaches take no account of the ways students currently use digital technologies to learn about food, their bodies, or their health. Therefore, it is imperative that we begin to facilitate and document alternative, student-led ways of using digital technology in HPE.

It is now widely acknowledged by scholars that much of the uptake of digital technology in schools is driven by commercial and political imperatives (Buckingham 2015; Selwyn 2010). This means that money, time, and energy is spent on acquiring, maintaining, and learning how to use technology that may not be appropriate or necessary in specific school contexts. By contrast, we argue that we need to develop programmes of research that seek to work within the conditions of possibility that exist in schools. Rather than an exercise in identifying what technology schools lack or 'need', we need to begin with the strengths of local educational communities and infrastructures. A programme of research that begins with the concrete realities and the strengths of schools will be significant for educational policy because it will connect local conditions with pedagogical practice and produce knowledge about how existing digital resources can be employed for educationally innovative purposes.

In simple terms, what we are proposing is that we think about learning in HPE in a way that transcends both the top-down approach of public health and the transmission models of learning that have long dominated HPE practice (Kirk 2010). In fact, the field of HPE does not yet have a robust evidence base on which to base student-centred pedagogies that leverage the educational experiences digital technology makes available. This would be innovative work because it will need to bring learning theories developed for and through digital technology to bear on HPE for the first time.

Much more work needs to be done to gain insight into the limits and possibilities of using digital technologies to develop relevant and student-driven ways of teaching HPE in schools. Research that builds knowledge about how and why young people use digital technologies to construct HPE-related knowledge is necessary. This 'new' knowledge can then be used to create new democratic pedagogical frameworks and practices that prioritise student engagement and student voice. While the data set on which this book is based offers some answers to the question of how and why young people use digital technologies to find health-related knowledge, this and other questions inspired by the construction of this chapter deserve our serious attention:

1   How and why do young people use digital technologies to find health and movement related knowledge?
2   What are the constraints and enablers involved in co-constructing relevant digital HPE pedagogies with young people?
3   How can we (teachers, students, school leaders, researchers) expand the pedagogical possibilities available to HPE teachers?

Youth participatory action research

Pursuing the answers to the above questions means forging sustainable partnerships with students and teachers in schools. Youth Participatory Action Research (YPAR) is a systematic approach for engaging young people in transformational educational experiences that could support such work. YPAR researchers accept that expertise and knowledge are widely distributed, and recognise that young people have the expertise, capacity, and agency to analyse and transform their social and educational contexts (Cammarota and Fine 2008; Enright and O'Sullivan 2010b, 2012, 2013). More important, however, YPAR assumes that it is through adults and young people working *together* that democratic and relevant educational practice will be constructed and advanced (Enright and O'Sullivan 2010a; Ginwright 2008). Philosophically, YPAR is based on Friere's (1993) notion of praxis-critical reflection and action. In the context of what we are proposing in this chapter, this means producing knowledge and action *with* students in order to generate new insights and move HPE practice and policy forward.

YPAR could be used to engage students in a collaborative process of HPE curricular construction that uses digital technology as its primary pedagogical tool. However, unlike most previous YPAR work in education and in HPE in particular, we argue there is a necessity to move away from deficit-based discourses and the preoccupation with changing behaviours in order to solve problems. Instead, we need to generate 'appreciative' insights (Enright *et al.*

2014; Ghaye *et al.* 2008) into what supports and enables engaging and sustainable pedagogical innovation. Therefore, as well as aligning with a 'strengths-based' philosophy, this research and pedagogical agenda would harness students' interests and talents, in addition to their health, movement, and technological expertise (Enright and Gard 2015; Kenway and Bullen 2008).

In the interests of sustainable educational change and forging collaborative relationships across institutional boundaries, the expertise teachers bring to the YPAR process would, of course, also be recognised as integral to this kind of praxis. Much has been written about teachers' lack of technological expertise in the context of increasing pressure to understand and use digital technologies to foster more authentic digital learning (Buckingham 2013). Yet, this literature often overlooks the skills and knowledge of students that teachers bring to any pedagogical encounter. In keeping with one of the fundamental tenets of YPAR, therefore, teachers would play a central role in this research and pedagogical innovation as gate-keepers, supporters, informants, conduits, and co-researchers.

Summary of key messages

- We need to work to create alternative, student-led ways of using digital technologies in HPE. It is through adults and young people working *together* that democratic and relevant educational practice will be constructed and advanced.
- Rather than an exercise in identifying what skills, knowledge, expertise, or resources students, teachers, and schools lack or 'need', we should begin with the strengths of these stakeholders and their local educational communities and infrastructures.
- It is now widely acknowledged by scholars that much of the uptake of digital technology in schools is driven by commercial and political imperatives. This means that money, time, and energy is spent on acquiring, maintaining, and learning how to use technology that may not be appropriate or necessary in specific school contexts. By contrast, we advocate working within the conditions of possibility that pertain to individual schools, connecting local conditions with pedagogical practice and producing knowledge about how existing digital resources can be employed for educationally innovative purposes.

Notes

1 We use the term digital technologies in quite a broad sense to refer to computer hardware and software, digital media, devices and systems, contemporary and emerging communication technologies, and so on.
2 In Australia, health and physical education (HPE) is the name of the learning area/ subject which has as one of its aims 'to enable students to access, evaluate and synthesise information to take positive action to protect, enhance and advocate for their own and others' health, wellbeing, safety and physical activity participation across their lifespan' (ACARA 2017).

3　As we worked to revise this chapter, the Facebook and Cambridge Analytica data harvesting revelations became global news. One headline reads 'Facebook is killing democracy with its personality profiling data' (Summers 2018). This scandal is, among other things, another reminder that digital technologies can also be a threat to democracy.

4　Digital Literacy is a contested concept. However, the majority of definitions acknowledge it requires multiple skills (technical, cognitive, emotional), and manifests as the ability to use digital technologies to find, evaluate, create, and communicate information, and participate in the knowledge society effectively (Buckingham 2010; Alkali and Amichai-Hamburger 2004).

5　eHealth literacy has been defined as the use of emerging information and communications technology to improve or enable health and health care (Neter and Brainin 2012).

References

Ackard, D.M. and Neumark-Sztainer, D., 2001. Health care information sources for adolescents: Age and gender differences on use, concerns, and needs. *Journal of Adolescent Health*, 29(3), 170–176.

Alkali, Y. E. and Amichai-Hamburger, Y., 2004. Experiments in digital literacy. *CyberPsychology & Behavior*, 7(4), 421–429.

Asthana, S., 2009. Young people, new media, and participatory design. *In:* K. Tyner, ed., *Media Literacy: New Agendas in Communication*. Texas: College of Communication, 11–28.

Australian Bureau of Statistics., 2017. *Internet Activity.* Available from www.abs.gov.au/ausstats/abs@.nsf/mf/8153 (accessed 2 March 2018).

Beck, F., Richard, J.B., Nguyen-Thanh, V., Montagni, I., Parizot, I., and Renahy, E., 2014. Use of the internet as a health information resource among French young adults: Results from a nationally representative survey. *Journal of Medical Internet Research*, 16(5), 1–5.

Becker, T., 1998. Governance and electronic innovation: A clash of paradigms. *Information, Communication and Society*, 1(3), 339–343.

Bernstein, J., 2004. *Oppenheimer: Portrait of an enigma.* Chicago: Ivan R. Dee.

Bessant, J., 2014. *Democracy Bytes: New Media, New Politics and Generational Change.* London: Springer.

Buckingham, D., 2015. Do we really need media education 2.0? Teaching media in the age of participatory culture. *In:* T. Lin, V. Chen and C.S. Chai, eds., *New Media and Learning in the 21st Century*. Singapore: Springer, 9–21.

Buckingham, D., 2010. Defining digital literacy. *Nordic Journal of Digital Literacy*, 3(12), 59–71.

Buckingham, D. (2013) *Beyond Technology: Children's Learning in the Age of Digital Culture*, London: John Wiley & Sons.

Buckingham, D., 2008. *Youth, Identity, and Digital Media.* Cambridge, MA: MIT Press.

Buckingham, D. and Willett, R., 2013. *Digital Generations: Children, Young People, and the New Media.* London: Routledge.

Burns, J.M., Davenport, T.A., Durkin, L.A., Luscombe, G.M., and Hickie, I.B., 2010. The internet as a setting for mental health service utilisation by young people. *The Medical Journal of Australia*, 192(11), S22–6.

Cammarota, J. and Fine, M., 2008. *Revolutionizing Education: Youth Participatory Action Research in Motion.* New York: Routledge.

Castells, M., 1997. *The Power of Identity.* Oxford: Blackwell.

Coll, L., O'Sullivan, M., and Enright, E., 2018. The trouble with normal: (Re) imagining sexuality education with young people. *Sex Education*, 18(2), 157–171.

Cummiskey, M., 2011. There's an app for that smartphone use in health and physical education. *Journal of Physical Education, Recreation & Dance*, 82(8), 24–30.

Dahlberg, L., 2011. Re-constructing digital democracy: An outline of four 'positions'. *New Media & Society*, 13(6), 855–872.

Dahlgren, P., 2009. *Media and Political Engagement*. Cambridge: Cambridge University Press.

Diamond, L., 2010. Liberation technology. *Journal of Democracy*, 21(3), 69–83.

Enright, E., 2013. Young people as curators of physical culture: A metaphor to teach and research by. *In:* L. Azzarito and D. Kirk, eds., *Physical Culture, Pedagogies and Visual Methods*. London: Routledge, 198–211.

Enright, E. and Gard, M., 2015. Media, digital technology and learning in sport: A critical response to Hodkinson, Biesta and James. *Physical Education and Sport Pedagogy*, 21(1), 40–60.

Enright, E., Hill, J., Sandford, R., and Gard, M., 2014. Looking beyond what's broken: Towards an appreciative research agenda for physical education and sport pedagogy. *Sport, Education and* Society, 19(7), 912–926.

Enright, E., Robertson, J., Hogan, A., and Stylianou, M., 2016. The promise and messy realities of digital technology in physical education. *In:* A. Casey, V. Goodyear, and K. Armour, eds., *Digital Technologies and Learning in Physical Education: Pedagogical Cases*. London: Routledge, 173–190.

Enright, E. and O'Sullivan, M., 2012. Physical education 'in all sorts of corners': Student activists transgressing formal physical education curricular boundaries. *Research Quarterly for Exercise and Sport*, 83(2), 255–267.

Enright, E. and O'Sullivan, M., 2010a. 'Can I do it in my pyjamas?': Negotiating a physical education curriculum with teenage girls. *European Physical Education Review*, 16(3), 203–222.

Enright, E. and O'Sullivan, M., 2010b. Carving a new order of experience' *with* young people in physical education: Participatory action research as a pedagogy of possibility. *In:* M. O'Sullivan and A. MacPhail, eds., *Young People's Voices in Physical Education and Youth Sport*. London: Routledge, 163–185.

Eshet-Alkalai, Y., 2004. Digital literacy: A conceptual framework for survival skills in the digital era. *Journal of Educational Multimedia and Hypermedia*, 13(1), 93–106.

Eysenbach, G., 2008. Medicine 2.0: Social networking, collaboration, participation, apomediation, and openness. *Journal of Medical Internet Research*, 10(3), e22.

Ferrara, E., 2017. Measuring social spam and the effect of bots on information diffusion in social media. Available from: *arXiv preprint arXiv:1708.08134* (accessed 2 March 2018).

Freeman, J.L., Caldwell, P.H., Bennett, P.A., and Scott, K.M., 2018. How adolescents search for and appraise online health information: A systematic review. *The Journal of Pediatrics*, iFirst Article.

Freire, P., 1993. *Pedagogy of the Oppressed*. New York: Continuum.

Frith, E., 2017. *Social Media and Children's Mental Health: A Review of the Evidence*. Available from https://epi.org.uk/wp-content/uploads/2018/01/Social-Media_Mental-Health_EPI-Report.pdf (accessed 2 March 2018).

Fullagar, S., Rich, E. and Francombe-Webb, J., 2017. New kinds of (ab) normal?: Public pedagogies, affect, and youth mental health in the digital age. *Social Sciences*, 6(3), 99–112.

Gard, M., 2014. eHPE: A history of the future. *Sport, Education and Society*, 19(6), 827–845.

Gard, M. and Enright, E., 2016. Computer says no: An analysis of three digital food education resources. *Asia-Pacific Journal of Health, Sport and Physical Education*, 7(3), 205–218.

Gard, M., Hickey-Moody, A., and Enright, E., 2013. Youth culture, physical education and the question of relevance: After 20 years, a reply to Tinning and Fitzclarence. *Sport, Education and Society*, 18(1), 97–114.

Gard, M. and Pluim, C., 2014. *Schools and Public Health: Past, Present, Future*. New York: Lexington Books.

Ghaye, T., Melander-Wikman, A., Kisare, M., Chambers, P., Bergmark, U., Kostenius, C., and Lillyman, S., 2008. Participatory and appreciative action and reflection (PAAR) – democratizing reflective practices. *Reflective Practice*, 9(4), 361–397.

Ginwright, S., 2008. Collective Radical Imagination. *In:* J. Cammarota and M. Fine, eds., *Revolutionizing Education: Youth Participatory Action Research in Motion*. New York: Routledge, 13–22.

Goodyear, V.A., Armour, K.M. and Wood, H., 2018. Young people and their engagement with health-related social media: new perspectives. *Sport, Education and Society*, iFirst Article.

Gould, A.W. and Mazzeo, J., 1982. Age and sex differences in early adolescent's information sources. *The Journal of Early Adolescence*, 2(3), 283–292.

Gray, N.J., Klein, J.D., Noyce, P.R., Sesselberg, T.S., and Cantrill, J.A., 2005. Health information-seeking behaviour in adolescence: The place of the internet. *Social Science and Medicine*, 60(7), 1467–1478.

Hague, B. and Loader, B., 1999. *Digital Democracy: Discourse and Decision Making in the Information Age*. London: Routledge.

Hausmann, J.S., Touloumtzis, C., White, M.T., Colbert, J.A. and Gooding, H.C., 2017. Adolescent and young adult use of social media for health and its implications. *Journal of Adolescent Health*, 60(6), 714–719.

Hindman, M., 2008. *The Myth of Digital Democracy*. Princeton: Princeton University Press.

International Telecommunications Union., 2013. *Measuring the Information Society*. Available from www.itu.int/en/ITU-D/Statistics/Documents/publications/mis2013/MIS 2013_without_Annex_4.pdf (accessed 2 March 2018).

Kahne, J., Middaugh, E., and Allen, D., 2015. Youth, new media, and the rise of participatory politics. *In:* D. Allen and J. Light, eds., *From Voice to Influence: Understanding Citizenship in a Digital Age*. Chicago: University of Chicago Press, 35–56.

Kenway, J. and Bullen, E., 2008. The global corporate curriculum and the young cyberflaneur as global citizen. *In:* N. Dolby and F. Rizvi, eds., *Youth Moves: Identities and Education in Global Perspective*. New York: Routledge, 17–32.

Kirk, D., 2010. *Physical Education Futures*. London: Routledge.

Leahy, D., Burrows, L., McCuaig, L., Wright, J., and Penney, D., 2015. *School Health Education in Changing Times: Curriculum, Pedagogies and Partnerships*. London: Routledge.

Liao, P.A., Chang, H.H., Wang, J.H. and Sun, L.C., 2016. What are the determinants of rural-urban digital inequality among schoolchildren in Taiwan? Insights from Blinder-Oaxaca decomposition. *Computers and Education*, 95(1), 123–133.

Loader, B.D. and Mercea, D., 2011. Networking democracy? Social media innovations and participatory politics. *Information, Communication and Society*, 14(6), 757–769.

Lupton, D., 2013. Quantifying the body: Monitoring and measuring health in the age of mHealth technologies. *Critical Public Health*, 23(4), 393–403.

Mitchell, K.J., Ybarra, M.L., Korchmaros, J.D., and Kosciw, J.G., 2014. Accessing sexual health information online: Use, motivations and consequences for youth with different sexual orientations. *Health Education Research*, 29(1), 147–157.

Montgomery, K.C., 2008. Youth and digital democracy: Intersections of practice, policy, and the marketplace. *In:* W. L. Bennett, ed., *The John D. and Catherine T. MacArthur Foundation Series on Digital Media and Learning. Civic Life Online: Learning how Digital Media can Engage Youth*, Cambridge, MA: MIT Press, 25–49.

Neter, E. and Brainin, E., 2012. eHealth literacy: Extending the digital divide to the realm of health information. *Journal of Medical Internet Research*, 14(1), e19.

Pariser, E., 2011. *The Filter Bubble: How the New Personalized Web is Changing What We Read and How We Think*. London: Penguin.

Rich, E. and Miah, A., 2017. Mobile, wearable and ingestible health technologies: Towards a critical research agenda. *Health Sociology Review*, 26(1), 84–97.

Roberts-Holmes, G., 2014. Playful and creative ICT pedagogical framing: A nursery school case study. *Early Child Development and Care*, 184(1), 1–14.

Sanders, M. and George, A., 2017. Viewing the changing world of educational technology from a different perspective: Present realities, past lessons, and future possibilities. *Education and Information Technologies*, 22(6), 2915–2933.

Sefton-Green, J., 2004. *Digital Diversions: Youth Culture in the Age of Multimedia*. London: Routledge.

Selwyn, N., 2010. *Schools and Schooling in the Digital Age: A Critical Analysis*. London: Routledge.

Smeets, E., 2005. Does ICT contribute to powerful learning environments in primary education? *Computers and Education*, 44(3), 343–355.

Stern, N., 2007. *The Economics of Climate Change: The Stern Review*. Cambridge: Cambridge University Press.

St. Jean, B., Subramaniam, M., Taylor, N.G., Follman, R., Kodama, C., and Casciotti, D., 2015. The influence of positive hypothesis testing on youths' online health-related information seeking. *New Library World*, 116(3/4), 136–154.

Summers, T., 2018. Facebook is killing democracy with its personality profiling data. *The Conversation*. Available from https://theconversation.com/facebook-is-killing-democracy-with-its-personality-profiling-data-93611 (accessed 22 March 2018).

Swist, T., Collin, P., McCormack, J., and Third, A., 2015. *Social Media and the Well-being of Children and Young People: A Literature Review*. Prepared for the Commissioner for Children and Young People, Western Australia, Perth.

Third, A., Bellerose, D., De Oliveira, J.D., Lala, G., and Theakstone, G., 2017. *Young and Online: Children's Perspectives on Life in the Digital Age*. Sydney: Western Sydney University.

Vander Shee, C. and Boyles, D., 2010. Exergaming, corporate interests and the crises discourse of childhood obesity. *Sport, Education and Society*, 15(2), 169–185.

Wartella, E., Rideout, V., Montague, H., Beaudoin-Ryan, L., and Lauricella, A., 2016. Teens, health and technology: A national survey. *Media and Communication*, 4(3), 13–23.

Waasdorp, T.E. and Bradshaw, C.P., 2015. The overlap between cyberbullying and traditional bullying. *Journal of Adolescent Health*, 56(5), 483–488.

Part III

Evidence-based guidelines, recommendations, and actions

16 Right message, right time

How adults can support young people's engagement with health-related social media

Victoria A. Goodyear and Kathleen M. Armour

Chapter overview

Many relevant adults who are invested in young people's health and wellbeing (including teachers, parents/guardians, health professionals/practitioners, policy makers) are aware that young people are prolific users of social media, but they are uncertain about how to support young people in their engagement with health-related digital media. In this chapter, we review the evidence presented in the previous chapters and provide evidence-based guidance for educators, policy, and researchers. We consider clear challenges in the process of meeting the needs of multiple stakeholders and knowledge translation, and evaluate the effectiveness of the pedagogical case model as a professional development tool.

Introduction

In today's media-rich, technologically innovative environment, schools, teachers, parents, and carers are expected to ensure that young people remain healthy and safe online (Armour 2014; Harris *et al.* 2016; Livingstone *et al.* 2017; Patton *et al.* 2016). This places considerable pressure on contemporary adults who may be ill-equipped to meet young people's needs and demands in an increasingly complex digital media landscape (Livingstone *et al.* 2017; Livingstone and Third 2017). Indeed, many adults are struggling to keep track of the pace of technological advancement and the ways in which digital/online spaces – such as social media – are creating new ways of living and being for young people (Ito *et al.* 2010; Turkle 2017).

The contemporary digital world differs greatly to the childhood experiences of most adults (Buckingham 2013), and this has inevitably created challenges for the ways in which policy makers, schools, health and education professionals/practitioners, and parents and carers tend to frame and approach the types of support that they attempt to provide for young people (Clark 2013). It has been argued that adults tend to make judgements based on their childhood experiences of passive media (e.g. magazines or TV) (Clark 2013), and while there are some similarities between 'old' and 'new' media, adults can find that they lack the knowledge and skills they need to be able to understand and engage effectively with young people's digital spaces (boyd 2014; Livingstone *et al.* 2017), as a range of international evidence illustrates (see Kidron and Rudkin 2017; Third *et al.* 2014). At the very least, this suggests that policy makers, schools, health and education professionals/practitioners, and parents and carers need access to appropriate levels of professional support and the latest evidence-based guidance (Goodyear *et al.* 2018a, 2018b). While a gap between the worlds of adults and young people has always existed, and is apparent in contexts that transcend digital media, there appear to be very large gaps in adults' understanding of young people and their engagement with digital media, and this is creating problems for how young people are supported to grow and develop into healthy, knowledgeable, and safe citizens (Livingstone *et al.* 2017; Kidron and Rudkin 2017).

The aim of this book was to provide practical information for policy makers, schools, health and education practitioners/professionals, and researchers, as well as ensuring that the evidence presented would be engaging and relevant to parents/guardians. The focus has been on young people's engagement with health-related social media as one illustrative example of a very powerful digital health-related medium within the vast and expanding digital landscape. We adopted and adapted a pedagogical case model to structure the book in order to communicate evidence-based research in an accessible format and to position the book as a professional learning mechanism and resource. The book relies heavily on the perspectives and experiences of young people to frame analysis, discussion, and commentary.

The structure of the book reflects our ambitions. In Part I, we presented a series of data-rich case studies that illustrated some of the many ways in which young people engage with social media and how and why this can have an influence on their health-related knowledge, understanding, and behaviours. In Part II, we stepped back from the vivid data and drew on a range of different disciplinary perspectives to better understand the ways in which health-related social media can influence young people. In this third part, the information from the previous sections has been crystallised into evidence-based actions and guidelines that can help relevant adults to mitigate against risks while simultaneously optimising the potential for young people's engagement with digital health-related media. The purpose of this chapter is to answer the question: so what? Have we achieved what we and our chapter authors set out to do? Will the book be 'useful' to intended audiences and what are the barriers? We address these questions in four sections:

- Key findings: Meeting the needs of multiple stakeholders.
- Issues to be considered in the processes of knowledge creation, co-construction, and translation.
- A review of the effectiveness of the pedagogical cases model as a professional development tool.
- Where next?

Meeting the needs of multiple stakeholders

The chapters in this book have reinforced, vividly, the need to engage all health and wellbeing stakeholders if young people are to be supported to use digital media effectively. In particular, Part II provides evidence that the support young people require crosses multiple contexts (e.g. home, school, community settings, and digitally/online) and should involve diverse individuals (e.g. teachers, clinicians, social media site providers, peers). It was also apparent that there is a need for seamless support, and that a consistent message and approach must be adopted between different individuals, contexts, and sectors. There is robust evidence from other areas, such as in youth mental health, that the adoption of consistent messaging by policymakers, service providers, and schools is most likely to result in positive impacts on knowledge, understandings, and behaviours (Beidas *et al.* 2016; Patton *et al.* 2016). The main evidence-based message for stakeholders from this book can, therefore, be summarised as follows:

> Social media is a very powerful educative health resource that has considerable significance in the lives of contemporary young people. Most young people experience positive impacts and are critically aware users and generators of health-related social media. While the health-related risks of social media should not be excluded, adults must focus on supporting young people to engage with social media so that they can realise more of the positive impacts on their health and wellbeing. The health-related risks of social media should not be ignored, but an action for adults is to become suitably digital literate so that they can promote positive outcomes and offer support to young people at times of vulnerability.

Although consistent messaging is important, it is also important to develop audience-specific messages (Holt *et al.* 2017; Perrier and Ginis 2018), whether that is for adult stakeholders or young people (Armour *et al.* 2017). To ensure the evidence presented in this book is useful, therefore, there is a need to consider what messages are relevant and to whom?

It has been challenging to identify the types of messages that are most relevant to different adult stakeholder groups. In the research, while there was some appreciation of difference between different groups of adults, such as teachers, researchers, or clinicians (see Chapters 2, 7, 10, 14), adults were mostly referred to as a homogenous group. In Part II, for example, there was little appreciation of different types of needs, priorities, knowledge, and skills that policy makers, teachers, health and education practitioners/professionals, and researchers may have. As a result, it has been challenging to develop audience-specific messages, as has been found elsewhere (Perrier and Ginis 2018). In contrast, authors throughout the book have been very clear that young people have very different experiences of social media and require different forms of support.

In this part, we draw upon all the evidence presented in the book in an attempt to identify the core messages that are relevant to different stakeholder groups, including policy makers, schools, health and education practitioners/ professionals, and researchers, and we then translate these messages into practical actions that could be taken by them. Building on theories of change, evidence-based presentation models, and communication frameworks (see Bryne, Albright, and Kardefelt-Winther 2016), our messages are communicated by identifying: (i) the specific contextual issues that are relevant to each stakeholder group; (ii) the main evidence-based message; and (iii) what actions the stakeholders could take.

Policy makers

Context

Policies in Europe are gradually shifting from a focus on a 'safer' engagement to a 'better' engagement with the internet (Bryne, Albright, and Kardefelt-Winther 2016) and there is a growing emphasis on education and the promotion of digital literacy in schools (Third *et al.* 2014). Yet, policies often fail to meet desired standards (Bryne, Albright, and Kardefelt-Winther 2016; Third *et al.*, 2014). There tends to be an overwhelming focus on risk-management and little guidance is currently available for schools, teachers, parents, and carers on how to ensure young people realise positive impacts from their engagement with digital media (Kidron and Rudkin 2017; Third *et al.* 2017). This issue is further compounded because relevant policies are scattered across a number of different sectors, such as education, ICT, cybersecurity, violence and abuse, where they use different evidence and the advice offered is often contradictory (Bryne, Albright, and Kardefelt-Winther 2016).

Evidence-based message

Policy has an important role to play in shaping the narratives that surround young people, social media, and health. It is vital that society becomes more aware of the range of positive health benefits that young people can gain from social media engagement, and acknowledge young people's existing critical skills. Risks should not be ignored, but the detail needs to be better understood and claims about risk need to be more evidence-based. Policy makers should, therefore, ensure that guidance, support, and training are provided for schools/ teachers and parents/guardians, and that it is accessible and based on the latest evidence. This also requires a level of quality assurance in order to navigate the plethora of programmes made available to schools on current issues related to health and wellbeing.

Actions

It is imperative that young people's health-related uses of social media are considered alongside policy issues related to internet safety, including sexting and cyberbullying. This includes an acknowledgement of digital health as a specific behaviour, where health-related knowledge, understandings, and behaviours can be shaped by social media. Evidence-based guidelines and resources should be created for service providers of social media and for schools and teachers, and parents, and carers, detailing how young people could be empowered and supported to use social media for positive health education. Guidance should also include direction for how schools and teachers and parents and carers manage risk and pathways of further professional digital health support should be addressed when negative impacts arise. Training funds need to be allocated to schools to support teacher professional learning about social media, and to ensure that schools and teachers can engage with the latest evidence-based practices. Policy makers should also engage in conversations with young people, to ensure that policies remain current and reflective of young people's uses and experiences of digital media.

Schools

Context

Schools offer a primary site from which to reach a large number of young people, and they are contexts where high-quality health education can be provided for young people (Patton *et al.*, 2016). Many schools across international contexts have taken a proactive role in supporting young people's health and ensuring that they can use and engage with the internet responsibly and effectively (Leahy *et al.* 2016). There are numerous examples of effective school-wide policies on health and e-safety; for example, Chapter 13 refers to the Australian context and a recent focus in schools on the development of health literacy. Schools can also make proactive links with the wider community, and this has been shown to be beneficial in engaging parents and other health and wellbeing professionals in the support that can be offered to young people (see Chapter 10).

Evidence-based message

Schools should take responsibility for providing an appropriate level of education on digital health for young people, teachers, and learning support staff. Schools could actively shape values, narratives, and discourses that outline how social media can be used by young people to promote their physical activity, improve their diet/nutritional behaviours, and strengthen understandings about body image perceptions (see Chapters 7, 8, 9, and 12). The issue of potential risk should not be ignored; instead educative approaches should be adopted in order to meet young people's demands and needs, rather than resorting to the 'banning' of devices in school settings (see Chapter 7). There are strong suggestions that digital education could be incorporated more effectively into both the pastoral system and the physical education curriculum (see Chapters 8, 9, and 12) and that teachers are an important source of support for young people (Chapter 7).

Actions

Headteachers should ensure that teachers can access appropriate and evidence-based forms of professional development or training to help them to deliver appropriate forms of digital health education to young people. Professional development and training should focus on supporting teachers and support staff to become digitally literate. This would help teachers to critically evaluate the relevance of health-related information for their own and young people's lives, as well as developing the digital skills to navigate social media so they can understand and offer appropriate levels of support to young people. Policies and curricula should be introduced in schools focused on digital health, and these could emphasise the positive ways in which social media can influence health. Direction is also required on how young people can access support if they feel vulnerable at a particular time point. Schools should ensure that there are sufficient opportunities for young people to be actively involved in the design of school-based initiatives, educational forms of support, and school-wide policies, and they should engage with external health and wellbeing professionals who can offer expert advice and curriculum support.

Health and education professionals/practitioners

Context

Health and education professionals/practitioners – such as physical education teachers, youth sport coaches, and/or external professional development providers – rarely have access to the latest evidence-based knowledge and practices (Armour *et al.* 2017; Griffiths, Armour, and Cushion 2018; Makopoulou 2018), particularly when it comes to digital technologies and social media (Casey, Goodyear, and Armour 2016). There is also evidence that engagement with professional development related to digital health-related media is limited, and there is very little guidance available on social media and its links to health (Chapter 9). In the context of physical education, it has been reported that teachers find it challenging to understand how best to integrate technology into their classrooms (Casey, Goodyear, and Armour 2016), and despite their enthusiasm, there is little robust guidance on the types of digital pedagogical practices that are more or less effective (Casey, Goodyear, and Armour 2017).

Evidence-based message

Digital health-related media is a potentially valuable learning resource for young people, especially where numerous sites and devices are used multiple times a day and are woven into the very fabric of contemporary youth culture (see Chapter 15).

In contrast to much risk-related rhetoric, young people report that digital health-related media can be a very powerful educative medium for them (see Chapters 2–7). As a result, the use of social media and other digital technologies could be harnessed by health and education professionals/practitioners to support the development of young people's health and wellbeing behaviours (see Chapter 9). For some young people, some of the time, they also require expert support from health and education professionals/practitioners, particularly at times of vulnerability and when they find themselves in situations that could result in harm (see Chapters 10 and 12). Health and education professionals/practitioners may find it helpful to note that young people regard this professional source of information as valuable (see Chapter 10) and there could be an enhanced supporting role for physical education teachers (see Chapter 9).

Actions

This book has been designed to act as a professional development tool for health and education professionals/practitioners. Parts I and II offer evidence of young people's diverse experiences of health-related social media, and this could be used to prompt critical enquiry and support the development of new practices. It is also clear that professionals/practitioners should promote young people's digital agency and engage in ongoing conversations to design relevant and effective practices that optimise the power of digital health-related media as a learning resource (Chapters 12 and 15). Activist approaches (Chapter 9) or strengths-based curricula (Chapters 8 and 15) are key ways in which young people can help adults to learn about the numerous ways in which they shape and are shaped by technology and the implications for developing effective educational support. Furthermore, these approaches – alongside body pedagogies (Chapters 8 and 12) – are key ways in which professionals/practitioners can harness young people's very specific levels of expertise in digital contexts.

Researchers

Context

In a wide range of fields, local and national governments and third sector providers contribute to the types of practices, programmes, or interventions that are adopted in schools, in homes, by families and/or within community settings (Bryne, Albright, and Kardefelt-Winther 2016). These powerful organisations often rely heavily on research to determine the types of guidance and support that are offered to adults and, in turn, young people (Bryne, Albright, and Kardefelt-Winther 2016; Holt *et al.* 2017; Livingstone *et al.* 2017), and this is certainly the case in health-related issues (Patton *et al.* 2016). Current research, however, has failed to offer different types of insights that can challenge, contradict, or even oppose the widely held opinion that social media is harmful for young people's health.

Evidence-based message

To date, understandings about young people's experiences of digital health-related media have been methodologically and conceptually constrained. The impacts of digital media on health and wellbeing behaviours have not been investigated in ways that provide rigorous outcomes, and there appears to be very limited robust evidence that identifies causal links between digital media engagement and positive or negative physical and mental health outcomes (see Przybylski and Weinstein 2017a, 2017b). These limitations are the result of research across numerous disciplines being dominated by a focus on the medium(s), and user/participant responses to pre-determined capabilities (e.g. accessibility/visibility of information or surveillance/control practices) (Miller *et al.* 2016). Data have also been drawn primarily from surveys, observations and/or parent perspectives, with a dominant focus on vulnerable youth and/or risky online behaviours (James 2014; Mascheroni, Jorge, and Farrugia 2014; Wartella *et al.* 2016). Conceptually, there are further limitations. Research tends to report on risks because it has been grounded in concepts of power, surveillance, governance, and risk (Chapter 12). As a result of these methodological and conceptual weaknesses, many existing programmes/interventions and/or policies tend to be ineffective, as they are based on little, poor, or outdated data that are reported out of context, and grounded in risk/negative outcomes (Gaplin and Taylor 2017).

Actions

There is an urgent need to develop a robust evidence-base that can explain young people's engagement with contemporary digital media, and how and why digital media engagement impacts on their health-related knowledge. This book has reported on data that provides new evidence on the intensity, complexity, and diversity of young people's engagement with social media. As these data show, young people are both critically engaged and also vulnerable users and generators of health-related content (see Chapters 2–7). Methodologically, and building on earlier research in the fields of anthropology, psychology, and sociology (see Chapter 1), we have reported on the value of using participatory methods to engage with young people's perspectives and experiences of digital media. Conceptually, and similar to Rich (see Chapter 12), we have also provided new insights into the importance of adopting a pedagogically informed approach in order to engage with young people's needs and understand how their knowledge and behaviours are influenced. The framework presented in Chapter 1, although 'tentative', is an attempt to offer an advanced conceptualisation of pedagogy that is driven by content, and that can be used in future research to shift the narrative away from an overbearing focus on risk. In Part II, a range of theories are also explained, that can provide new ways of understanding health and young people's engagement with digital technologies. Further empirical evidence is, however, required. In particular, we suggest that research should engage with young people's agency and develop new methodological, conceptual, and ethical techniques that can explain how and why young people, from varying contexts, shift from being critical and effective users of social media to vulnerable and potentially at risk.

In summary, the data and analyses presented in this book offer some important and practical advice for different stakeholders. Yet, the translation of research into effective practice has always been challenging. In the next section, we explore these challenges to identify effective ways forward.

Issues to be considered in the processes of knowledge creation, co-construction, and translation

As we outlined in Chapter 1, in order to determine the types of support that young people require from adults, it is important to recognise that the perspectives of young people matter (Galpin and Taylor 2017; Third *et al.* 2017, 2014). Listening to young people is not only important for supporting their right to expression, but for understanding how their behaviours and knowledge are simultaneously shaping and being shaped by digital technologies (Third *et al.* 2017). Young people can provide insights into whether their health-related needs, hopes and wishes are being fulfilled and the role, or future role, of digital technology in supporting, hindering, and/or harnessing these needs (Third *et al.* 2017). Research that aims to generate insights into the ways in which young people use and experience social media, therefore, appears to be one way to ensure that the support offered to young people is more accommodating and reflective of their needs and demands. In short, we need to focus on the processes of knowledge creation, co-construction, and translation in order to meet the needs of all parties in this space.

Although generating evidence from the perspectives of young people is important, translating that research into evidence with which adults can engage and then use is equally important. Historically, it was thought that researchers simply had to conduct their research *on* 'subjects' and then deliver the research findings to relevant stakeholders who would act on the results (Grimshaw *et al.* 2012; Morden *et al.* 2015). It has since become apparent that this notion of translation is ineffective and, possibly, even unethical. In her AERA Presidential Address, Oakes (2017, p. 91) argued that 'engaging with publics to raise awareness of common problems is a central charge for researchers'. Oakes (2017) made the point that 'perceptions and politics don't change just because they conflict with the data' (p. 91). Scholars must be prepared to translate research in ways that 'effectively communicate research findings and recommendations to various publics in accessible and useful forms' (Oakes 2017, p. 98). Although in this research we have developed the research findings into user-friendly 'guidelines' (see Goodyear, Armour, and Wood 2018b), we also recognise Morden *et al.*'s (2015, p. 1560) point that 'the mere presence of guidelines, no matter how clearly communicated, is insufficient to change practice'. Certainly, novel ways are required to engage researchers and participants and to close persistent research-theory-practice gaps (Armour, 2017, 2014; Holt *et al.* 2017; Perrier and Ginis 2018).

While frameworks vary (Morden *et al.* 2015), knowledge translation refers to the process of translating research evidence into information that is delivered in a format appropriate for those who can make best use of it (Perrier and Ginis 2018). The process of knowledge translation is very dynamic and iterative, involving interactions between researchers and knowledge users that can improve the application of knowledge to provide more effective policies, programmes and practices (Morden *et al.* 2015; Perrier and Ginis 2018). Collaborating with stakeholders throughout the research is therefore a critical element of knowledge translation and is a process that facilitates the integrity of guidelines, practices, policies, and/or interventions (Holt *et al.* 2017).

In the research that underpins this book we attempted to move beyond the transfer of information and toward an iterative and dynamic approach to knowledge translation. Young people and collaborations with key stakeholders were at the heart of this research design and its conduct. In this book, one of the strategies we used was the adoption of the 'pedagogical cases' model (Armour 2017, 2014) in order to bridge the multiple gaps we identified in the existing research, in the new data, and between disciplinary approaches. In Chapter 1, we defined this approach and explained how the pedagogical case model could bridge theory-research-practice gaps through offering a bank of case studies around which stakeholder learning could be organised. In short, pedagogical cases is a multi-disciplinary approach to knowledge translation, whereby academics from different disciplines analyse case studies of young people and/or teachers, with the intention of developing practical and pedagogical evidence-based actions that can better meet learners' diverse needs (Armour 2017).

In this book, we adapted and refined the pedagogical case model by: (i) *constructing* evidence-based composite narrative case studies from our funded research projects with over 1,300 young people; (ii) *co-constructing* case studies in a way that engaged with and presented the voices of both young people and key stakeholders (e.g. schools, teachers, physical activity and health leaders in community settings, and policy and industry professionals); and (iii) *translating* the research through the identification of evidence-based practical solutions and through different discipline-based analyses of the case study chapters. This refined approach enabled us to retain the centrality of young people's voices throughout the book.

We were also able to ensure that the disciplinary analyses and identification of practical solutions reflected young people's experiences of social media, as well as their contemporary demands and needs. Consistent with knowledge translation frameworks, the engagement of key stakeholders also offered a more rounded picture of young people's physical activity and health education, helping to ensure relevance to a wide audience, and with practical solutions that could be effective in a range of contexts and settings. The pedagogical case study model is therefore strongly grounded in the concept of knowledge translation. The aim of engaging iteratively and dynamically with young people and key stakeholders was to ensure that this book and the evidence it presents could engage adults and influence the ways in which they support young people's engagement with digital health-related media. It is acknowledged that delivering impact of this nature will require further and multi-layered engagement strategies over time.

A central component of knowledge translation is the evaluation of implementation evidence (Holt *et al.* 2017; Perrier and Ginnis 2018). To date, however, there is limited evidence on how the pedagogical case model as used previously has impacted the knowledge, understanding, or practices of key practitioners. In this book we are seeking to influence schools, teachers, physical activity and health leaders in community settings, and policy and industry professionals. Monitoring the impact trail, therefore, will allow us to reflect back on the wider pedagogical case model and its effectiveness. The question remains however as to whether the pedagogical case model is effective in 'getting the right message to the right people' and in a way that clearly outlines what *adults need to know, should do, and act on in order to support young people*. There is a large literature on influencing adults in the context of practitioners and professional development. In the following section, we provide an overview of this literature and this provides some important clues about how best to ensure that our knowledge translation ambitions are met.

A review of the pedagogical cases model as a professional development tool

In a range of fields, professional development is regarded as a central mechanism to support the development of professionals'/practitioners' knowledge, understanding, skills, and practices (Armour and Chambers 2014; Griffiths *et al.* 2018). Yet, in sport and exercise pedagogy, as in other fields, practitioners/professionals report that they rarely engage with the types of professional development activities that support their learning and/or are capable of supporting the development of their practices (Armour *et al.* 2017; Griffiths *et al.* 2018). The professional development offered by a range of trusts, organisations, and/or researchers is often less effective than designers anticipated.

To meet young people's demands and needs there is a clear need to ensure that practitioners/professionals have access to the most up-to-date evidence from a range of sub/disciplines (Armour 2017, 2014), and that a variety of methods, tools, and resources are deployed to support authentic learning (Tannehill, van der Mars, and MacPhail 2015). The function of professional development is typically grounded in this understanding, where professional development activities operate as a space or tool for the transfer of knowledge (Armour *et al.* 2017). In sport and exercise pedagogy it is evident that many professional development activities and/or courses focus on information-providing activities (Griffiths *et al.* 2018). Examples include workshops on a particular teaching method or practitioner-focused textbooks that provide step-by-step instructions on how to implement a model or framework to achieve particular outcomes, such as motivation. Similar to Morden *et al.*'s (2015) critique of guidelines, merely delivering knowledge to professionals/practitioners in workshops or via textbooks is insufficient to support practitioner/professional learning (Griffiths *et al.* 2018). Professional development conceptualised as knowledge *transfer* rather than exchange or translation is an approach that ignores practitioner/professional judgement, the needs of the local context and, importantly, the diverse needs of young people.

At one level, this book could be conceptualised as a knowledge-transfer tool or an evidence-giving activity. Through the lens of knowledge transfer, the book provides practitioners/professionals with access to the latest evidence-based thinking on a contemporary issue impacting on young people's health and well-being. Yet the pedagogical case model was not designed merely to transfer information 'to' key stakeholders to use in their contexts. Instead, the pedagogical case model has been designed to ensure that it acts as a learning resource for a range of stakeholders, and to prompt thinking, critical enquiry, and the development of appropriate practices by stakeholders in their respective contexts. The book is also 'open access', thereby overcoming the persistent issues associated with ensuring that research is accessible to professionals/practitioners (Armour 2014).

Although the evidence-base on the characteristics of effective professional development are inconclusive (Goodyear 2017), there is some agreement that professional development is most likely to support practitioner learning when it is content-rich, engaging, relevant, and sustained (Cordingly *et al.* 2015; Griffiths *et al.* 2018; Makopoulou 2018). Case studies were used, therefore, to ensure that the empirically rich evidence from the research is presented in a way that is engaging and relevant to a range of stakeholders. Certainly, an extensive evidence-base reports that case studies are an effective tool for professional development since they provide practitioners/professionals with 'real life' and 'contextualised' examples that can be taken forward into a range of contexts (Armour and Jones 1998; Connell 1986; Jones *et al.* 2003; Stenhouse 1980; Thomas 2011). To further support stakeholder learning, the case studies (Chapters 2–7) are structured in the format of composite, empirically rich narratives. Through narrative, research evidence is presented in a way that is understandable, more human, and more memorable (Smith *et al.* 2013). Furthermore, narratives can 'open up, rather than close down, different ways of being and possible worlds in a manner that provokes people to think with and not just about research' (Smith *et al.* 2013, p. 2047). Using empirically rich, composite narrative case studies is, therefore, a strategy designed to support stakeholder learning in order to close gaps between the ways in which adults and young people understand social media.

Characteristics of effective professional development also include concepts of agency and capacity building, whereby adult learners are prompted, encouraged, and supported to critically evaluate evidence, inquire into their practices, and develop new insights that are aligned with the needs of their own contexts (Armour *et al.* 2017; Cordingly *et al.* 2015; Griffiths *et al.* 2018). A focus on young people's different experiences – through six case studies – was also an important mechanism for informing adults in a way that they could offer challenges to simplistic and/or prescriptive approaches to supporting young people's health and wellbeing (Armour *et al.* 2017), such as the widely adopted and promoted regulatory advice currently given to many adults on young people's uses of social media (Livingstone *et al.* 2017). The aim was to report young people's diverse experiences in all their richness such that adults are supported to develop new insights and are prompted to consider the relevance of information presented in relation to the needs and demands of the young people for whom they are responsible.

Another important characteristic of effective professional development is its capacity to build connections between theory-research-practice. In this book, each section has aimed to bridge these theory-research-practice gaps. In Part I, evidence generated from young people was combined with the stakeholder analysis (that included a range of international multi-sector researchers, practitioners, and health and wellbeing professionals), and evidence and analysis were combined to provide considerations for research, policy, and/or practice. In Part II, each of the multi-disciplinary chapter authors analysed the evidence-base case studies and identified the types of practices and/or interventions from their discipline that could support young people's engagement with digital health-related media. As a result, the structure of the chapters within Parts I and II has been designed to offer evidence-based and practice-referenced insights, suggestions, and recommendations on how a range of different stakeholders can support young people's engagement with digital health-related media. Drawing on literature in the fields of professional development and knowledge translation (Armour *et al.* 2017; Holt *et al.* 2017; Smith *et al.* 2013), this dynamic approach to theory-research-practice serves to ensure that a range of professionals/practitioners can engage with the evidence and translate the findings as appropriate in their contexts and settings.

What next?

There is a growing body of evidence reporting on the opportunities of digital/online environments to facilitate discussion, exchange, and dissemination between researchers, professional development facilitators, and key stakeholders (Carpenter and Krukta 2014). In the field of sport and exercise pedagogy, Massive Open Online Courses (Goodyear *et al.* 2017), Twitter chats (Goodyear *et al.* 2014) and blogs (Casey *et al.* 2014) have been evidenced as effective knowledge-exchange and professional development tools. Further, much could be learned from the experiences of young people that are presented in this book about how they interact and learn via social media. For many young people, there was evidence that engagement with social media is a seamless learning experience that binds online/offline contexts and allows young people to engage with the latest information. We, therefore, challenge academics to consider the types of knowledge-exchange activities they engage with, and how they can optimise the use of digital technologies and digital media to facilitate sustained debate and discussion. It would certainly be of interest to see how papers and symposia presented at international conferences build on knowledge from previous years, where there is potential for different sub/disciplines to develop thematic approaches to conference sessions.

We make no claim that the pedagogical cases model used in this book has addressed all the challenges of bridging research-theory-practice gaps in this field. Specifically, further analysis is required to synthesise the information generated from young people and key stakeholders (i.e. international multi-sector researchers, practitioners, and health and wellbeing professionals) (Part 1), and from the different disciplinary perspectives: health, physical education, eating disorders, human geography, and social capital, public pedagogies, memes, health literacy, and youth methodologies (Part II). There are also other disciplines that could provide helpful insights into the data and the analysis, and further stakeholder groups, such as parents, that could have extended our under-standings of the types of support for young people that will be effective.

Yet, this next phase of analysis will be most effective if it is undertaken in collaboration with key stakeholders in a knowledge-exchange framework and it is likely that this will generate further questions that will need to be investigated. As with much research, answers are often partial and tantalising, and they serve to generate more nuanced questions. For example: What are the tipping points when young people switch from being critical, effective users and generators of health-related content to potentially vulnerable and at risk?; What role do schools, family members, and peers play in influencing the health-related content young people engage with through digital media?; What do parents need to know and do? How can we effectively investigate young people's agency and explain how their digital cultures influence health-related knowledge and behavi-ours?; and What knowledge translation methods will be effective in helping adults and key stakeholders to engage with the evidence?

As a starting point for the next phase of this work, particularly in developing the pedagogical case model as a professional development tool and promoting knowledge-exchange, we encourage you to engage with us about this research via Twitter and our website. We acknowledge that social media and other digital platforms change over time but for the foreseeable future, we can engage with you through Twitter, email and our OpenCPD website:

Victoria A. Goodyear: @VGoodyear
Kathleen M. Armour: @ArmourKathy
Website: opencpd.net

References

Armour, K.M., 2017. Pedagogical cases: A new translational mechanism to bridge theory/research practice gaps in youth physical activity education (PAE). *Kinesiology Review*, 6(1), 42–50.

Armour, K.M., 2014. *Pedagogical Cases in Physical Education and Youth Sport*. London: Routledge.

Armour, K.M. and Chambers, F.C., 2014. 'Sport and exercise pedagogy'. The case for a new integrative sub-discipline in the field of sport and exercise sciences/kinesiology/ human movement sciences. *Sport, Education and Society*, 19, 855–868.

Armour, K.M. and Jones, R.L., 1998. *Physical Education Teachers' Lives and Careers: PE, Sport and Educational Status*. London: Routledge.

Armour, K.M., Quennerstedt, M., Chambers, F., and Makopoulou, K. 2017. What is 'effective' CPD for contemporary physical education teachers? A Deweyan framework. *Sport, Education and Society*, 22(7), 799–811.

Beidas, R.S., Stewart, R.E., Adams, D.R., Fernandez, T., Lustbader, S., Powell, B.J., Aarons, G.A., Hoagwood, K.E., Evans, A.C., Hurforf, M.O., Rubin, R., Hadley, T., Mandell, D.S., and Barg, F.K. 2016. A multi-level examination of stakeholder perspectives of implementation of evidence-based practices in a large urban publically-funded mental health system. *Administration and Policy in Mental Health and Mental Health Service Research*, 43(6), 893–908.

boyd, d., 2014. *It's Complicated: The Social Lives of Networked Teens*. London: Yale University Press.

Bryne, J., Albright, K., and Kardefelt-Winther, D., 2016. *Using Research Findings for Policy-Making*. London: Global Kids Online.

Buckingham, D., 2016. Is there a digital generation? *In:* D. Buckingham and R. Willett, eds., *Digital Generations: Children, Young People and the New Media*. London: Routledge, 1–18.

Carpenter, J.P. and Krukta, D.G., 2014. How and why educators use Twitter: A survey of the field. *Journal of Research on Technology in Education*, 46(4), 414–434.

Casey, A., Goodyear, V.A., and Armour, K.M., 2017. Rethinking the relationship between pedagogy, technology and learning in health and physical education. *Sport, Education and Society*, iFirst.

Casey, A., Goodyear, V.A., and Armour, K.A., 2016. *Digital Technologies and Learning in Physical Education: Pedagogical Cases*. London: Routledge.

Casey, A., Hill, J., and Goodyear, V.A., 2014. 'PE doesn't stand for physical education it stands for public embarrassment': Voicing experiences and proffering solutions to girls' disengagement in PE. *In:* S. Sanders, S. Flory, A. Tischler, eds., *Sociocultural Issues in Physical Education: Case Studies for Teachers*. London: Rowman & Littlefield, 37–53.

Clark, L.S., 2013. *The Parent App: Understanding Families in the Digital Age*. Oxford: Oxford University Press.

Connell, R.W., 1986. *Teachers' Work*. London: George, Allen & Unwin.

Cordingly, P., Higgins, S., Greany, T., Buckler, N., Coles-Jordan, D., Crisp, B., ... Coe, R., 2015. *Developing Great Teaching: Lessons from the International Reviews into Effective Professional Development*. London, UK: Teacher Development Trust.

Gaplin, A. and Taylor, G., 2017. Changing behaviour: Children, adolescents and screen use. Accessed from: www.bps.org.uk/sites/bps.org.uk/files/Policy%20-%20Files/Changing %20behaviour%20-%20children,%20adolescents,%20and%20screen%20use.pdf.

Goodyear, V.A., 2017. Sustained professional development on cooperative learning: Impact on six teachers' practices and students' learning. *Research Quarterly for Exercise and Sport*, 88(1), 83–94.

Goodyear, V.A., Armour, K.M., and Wood, H., 2018a. Young people and their engagement with health-related social media: New perspectives. *Sport, Education and Society*, iFirst.

Goodyear, V.A., Armour, K.M., and Wood, H., 2018b. *The Impact of Social Media on Young People's Health and Wellbeing: Evidence, Guidelines and Actions*. Birmingham, UK: University of Birmingham.

Goodyear, V.A., Griffiths, M., and Armour, K.M., 2017. Effective professional development for teachers and coaches: A new role for MOOCs?. Paper presented at the Physical Education and Health Conference Canada, St Johns, Canada.

Goodyear, V.A., Casey, A., and Kirk, D., 2014. Tweet me, message me, like me: Using social media to facilitate pedagogical change within an emerging community of practice. *Sport, Education and Society*, 19(7), 927–943.

Griffiths, M.A., Armour, K.M., and Cushion, C.J., 2018. 'Trying to get our message across': Successes and challenges in an evidence-based professional development programme for sport coaches. *Sport, Education and Society*, 23(3), 283–295.

Grimshaw, J.M., Eccles, M.P., Lavis, J.N., Hill, S.J., and Squires, J.E., 2012. Knowledge translation of research findings. *Implementation Science*, 7, 1–17.

Harris, J., Cale, L., Duncombe, R., and Musson, H., 2016. Young people's knowledge and understanding of health, fitness, and physical activity: Issues, divides and dilemmas. *Sport, Education and Society*, iFirst.

Holt, N.L., Camiré, M., Tamminen, K.A., Pankow, K., Pynn, S.R., Strachan, L., MacDonald, D.J., Fraser-Thomas, J. 2017. PYDSportNET: A knowledge translation project bridging gaps between research and practice in youth sport. *Journal of Sport Psychology in Action*, iFirst.

Ito, M., Baumer, S., Bittanti, M., boyd, d., Cody, R., *et al.*, 2010. *Hanging Out, Messing Around, and Geeking Out: Kids Living and Learning with New Media*. Cambridge, MA: MIT Press.

James, C., 2014. *Disconnected: Youth, New Media and the Ethics Gap*. London: MIT Press.

Jones, R.L., Armour, K.M., and Potrac, P., 2003. *Sports Coaching Cultures: From Practice to Theory*. London: Routledge.

Kidron, B. and Rudkin, A., 2017. Digital childhood: Addressing childhood development milestones in the digital environment. Accessed from: www.google.com/search?client =safari&rls=en&q=Digital+Childhood+Addressing+Childhood+Development+Milesto nes+in+the+Digital+Environment&ie=UTF-8&oe=UTF-8.

Leahy, D., Burrows, L., McCuaig, L., Wright, J., and Penney, D., 2016. *School Health Education in Changing Times*. London: Routledge.

Livingstone, S., Ólafsson, K., Helsper, E.J., Lupiàñez-Villanueva, F., Veltri, G.A., and Folkvord, F., 2017. Maximising opportunities and minimizing risks for children online: The role of digital skills in emerging strategies of parental mediation. *Journal of Communication*, 67(1), 82–105.

Livingstone, S. and Third, A., 2017. Children and young people's rights in the digital age: An emerging agenda. *New Media & Society*, 19(5), 657–670.

Makopoulou, K. 2018. An investigation into the complex process of facilitating effective professional learning: CPD tutors' practices under the microscope. *Physical Education and Sport Pedagogy*, 23(3), 250–266.

Mascheroni, G., Jorge, A., and Farrugia, L., 2014. Media representations and children's discourses on online risks: Findings from qualitative research in nine European countries. *Cyberpsychology: Journal of Psychosocial Research in Cyberspace*, 8(2), article 2.

Miller, D., Costa, E., Haynes, N., McDonald, T., Nicolescu, R., *et al.*, 2016. *How the World Changed Social Media*. London: UCL Press.

Morden, A., Ong, B.N., Brooks, L., Jinks, C., Porcheret, M., Edwards, J.J., and Dziedzic, K.S., 2015. Introducing evidence through research 'push': Using theory and qualitative methods. *Qualitative Health Research*, 25(11), 1560–1575.

Oakes, J., 2017. 2016 AERA presidential address. Public scholarship: Education research for a diverse democracy. *Educational Researcher*, 47(2), 91–104.

Patton, G.C., Sawyer, S.M., Santelli, J.S., Ross, D.A., Afifi, R. *et al.*, 2016. Our future: A Lancet commission on adolescent health and wellbeing. *Lancet*, 387, 2423–2478.

Perrier, M. and Ginis, K.A.M. 2018. Communicating physical activity information to people with physical disabilities. *In:* J.J.A. Dimmock and J. Compton, eds., *Persuasion and Communication in Sport, Exercise and Physical Activity*. Oxon: Routledge, 177–189.

Przybylski, A.K. and Weinstein, N., 2017a. Digital screen time limits and young children's psychological well-being: Evidence from a population-based study. *Child Development*, iFirst.

Przybylski, A.K. and Weinstein, N., 2017a. A large-scale test of the Goldilocks hypothesis: Quantifying the relations between digital-screen use and the mental well-being of adolescents. *Psychological Science*, 28(2), 204–215.

Smith, B., Papathomas, A., Ginis, K.A.M., and Latimer-Cheung, A.E., 2013. Understanding physical activity in spinal cord injury rehabilitation: Translating and communicating research through stories. *Disability and Rehabilitation*, 35(24), 2046–2055.

Stenhouse, L., 1980. Presidential Address: The study of samples and the study of cases. *British Educational Research Journal*, 6, 1, 1–6.

Tannehill, D., van der Mars, H., and MacPhail, A., 2015. *Building Effective Physical Education Programmes*. Burlington, MA: Jones and Bartlett Learning.

Third, A., Bellerose, D., Oliveira, J.D.D., Lala, G., and Theakstone, G., 2017. *Young and Online: Children's Perspectives On Life in the Digital Age*. Sydney: Western Sydney University.

Third, A., Bellerose, D., Dawkins, U., Keltie, E., and Pihl, K., 2014. *Children's Rights in the Digital Age: A Download from Children around the World*. Melbourne: Young and Well Cooperative Research Centre.

Thomas, G., 2011. *How To Do Your Case Study*. London, Sage.

Turkle S. 2017. *Alone Together: Why We Expect More from Technology and Less from Each Other*. 3rd Ed. New York: Basic Books.

Wartella, E., Rideout., V., Montague, H., Beaudoin-Ryan, and Lauricella, A., 2016. Teens, health, and technology: A national survey. *Media and Communications*, 4(3), 12–23.

17 Young people, social media, physical activity, and health

Final thoughts on the work, the present, and the future

Lorraine Cale

Chapter overview

It is a privilege to contribute the final chapter to this book which, as the previous chapters have illustrated, addresses an extremely important and much needed area of work. Whilst not focused on social media per se, my own research is concerned with the expression of health and the promotion of healthy, active lifestyles amongst young people, with the ultimate goal of enhancing their health. As evidenced throughout this book, social media and young people's interactions with social media are now so powerful and integral to this endeavour that they cannot be overlooked.

Introduction

In this chapter I offer an independent analysis and some closing reflections on the book and of the evidence, arguments, recommendations, and/or guidance presented in it. To begin, I outline what I perceive to be the major strengths of this work, before focusing on selected findings and common themes which struck me most on first reading, notably because they resonate and have parallels with my own health-related work as a researcher, a physical educator, and teacher educator. In my analysis, I cannot therefore help but be drawn largely to the findings, themes, and implications of relevance to the above and to the educational and school context. That said, the content equally applies to all adults with an interest in and responsibility for young people's health and well-being. To conclude the chapter, I comment on the future directions proposed for research and practice within the book and offer some further thoughts and suggestions relating to these, as appropriate.

The work

The strengths of this work are multiple. The book is clear, accessible, evidenced-based, and practical and, importantly, addresses empirical, methodological, and theoretical gaps in our understandings about young people's engagement with health-related social media. The aims of the book are clearly outlined in

Chapter 1, but in summary are concerned with increasing awareness of the impacts of social media on young people's health; generating new insights into young people's digital health and related behaviours; and informing new guidelines and actions for health and education. The book will thus be a valuable resource for health and education practitioners and other relevant adults including policy makers, researchers, and parents/guardians who are interested in supporting young people's health-related understandings and behaviours.

A key strength is the innovative research and rich and robust data upon which the book is based. These provide new and fascinating insights into young people's experiences of health-related social media and the reported impacts of this on their physical activity, health, and wellbeing. In this respect, the book highlights both health-related issues and opportunities associated with social media from young people's perspectives. The focus on issues *and* opportunities is arguably significant given the negative press, messages, and warnings often surrounding social media use, and overall it ensures a balanced and constructive approach to the area – a point I revisit later. The focus on young people's perspectives and experiences is also an important feature and strength. Hearing young people's voices in the case study chapters (Chapters 2–7) brings the book and content alive, with their accounts being hard hitting and concerning at times whilst encouraging and reassuring at others. Regardless of the emotions the case studies invoked, listening to, understanding, and responding to young people's experiences and working with them in so doing is crucial. I also return to this point later.

The approach to the book and to the research upon which it is based are furthermore novel. The adoption of co-constructed and participatory methods to generate the data on young people's social media experiences and the use of a 'content-led pedagogical framework' and 'pedagogical case model' approach to present, analyse, explain, and translate the data from multi-disciplinary stakeholders and academics is impressive and powerful. Lastly, the new evidence, the different theoretical insights, and practical guidelines resulting from this work should be instrumental in moving this important area forwards.

The present

The many perspectives and insights offered in this book provoked numerous thoughts and reflections I could explore but, as explained, I have been selective here. What is evident from the text though is that so many of the issues and challenges identified in relation to young people, social media, physical activity, and health equally apply to young people, physical activity and health more generally. They are, furthermore, issues which researchers, policy makers, and practitioners seem to have been grappling with for years. For example, issues concerning roles and responsibilities associated with health, the relative status of health, the nature and delivery of health and health-related knowledge, the validity of health messages and information, and health-related continuing professional development are widely reported in the literature. The difference is that when social media and health-related digital learning are added to the mix, the issues and challenges seem to be heightened. Conversely, and on a more optimistic note, the opportunities afforded by social media for physical activity and health should arguably also be heightened.

On the issue of roles and responsibilities, and as a physical educator and teacher educator, the reported absence of reference to physical education as a source of health education by the young people in the case studies is striking. This is particularly so given that health is an established goal of physical education in many countries and the subject often legitimises itself on this basis (Cale, Harris, and Duncombe 2016). Despite this finding, elsewhere young people have acknowledged teachers and physical education teachers to be important and reliable sources of health knowledge (Burrows 2010; Burrows and McCormack 2014; Harris *et al.* 2018; Hooper 2018), and encouragingly there was recognition by individuals in the case studies that physical education teachers are potentially a credible and important source of information and support (Chapters 7 and 9). However, the general omission of physical education in the young people's voices could be a 'wake up' call for the profession and it certainly suggests that the subject may not be at all influential in some young people's lives.

Of course, the above could partly be indicative of the status typically afforded to health in schools and physical education. Despite ever growing expectations on schools to promote health and physical activity (Cale *et al.* 2016), concerns have repeatedly been expressed over the relative marginal status and limited attention paid to these areas in practice (e.g. Alfrey, Cale, and Webb 2012; Cale, Harris, and Duncombe 2016; Harris 2010; Marks 2008; McMullen *et al.* 2015). For example, competing demands and pressures of academic accountability and results-driven curricula have been blamed for restricting the attention and time devoted to health and health-related activities in schools (Cardon *et al.* 2012; Larsen, Tjomsland, and Samdal 2013; Marks 2008). Whatever the reasons, if not addressed, this issue is likely to hinder progress and developments with regards social media, physical activity, and health in schools.

In addition, and arguably another indicator of the lower status afforded to health in schools is the long-standing and widely reported general absence of health from teachers' professional development profiles (Alfrey, Cale, and Webb 2012; Armour and Harris 2013; Cale, Harris, and Duncombe 2016; Castelli and Williams 2007; Jourdan *et al.* 2010; Kulinna *et al.* 2008; Larsen *et al.* 2013; Marks 2008; Speller *et al.* 2010). Evidence that there is also a lack of practitioner engagement with professional development related to health-related social media (Chapters 9 and 16) is, therefore, unsurprising. Perhaps also predictably, the above authors equally suggest that teachers, including physical education teachers, generally have limited knowledge and understanding of health.

The above issues undoubtedly raise questions concerning practitioners' 'preparedness' to adequately support and develop young people's health-related knowledge and behaviours (Alfrey *et al.* 2012; Cale, Harris, and Duncombe 2016). Given this, limitations in young people's health-related knowledge are to be expected and indeed have been found (e.g. Burrows 2008; Burrows, Wright, and McCormack 2009; Burrows and Wright 2010; Brusseau *et al.* 2011; Harris *et al.* 2018; Hooper 2018; Keating *et al.* 2009; Powell and Fitzpatrick 2015; Roth and Stamatakis 2010). Concurring with this literature, limited health knowledge and understandings are also evident among the young people in the case studies, for example, with confusion and/or misconceptions over FitTea (Chapter 2), 'no pain, no gain' exercise messages (Chapter 3), and health 'shortcuts' (Chapter 6).

It follows then that such shortcoming in teachers' and young people's health-related knowledge will influence both practice and decision-making with respect to physical activity and health. In teachers, this link has been acknowledged for some time (e.g. Alfrey, Cale, and Webb 2012; Castelli and Williams 2007; Harris and Leggett 2015; Hastie 2017; Kulinna *et al.* 2008; Keating *et al.* 2009; Puhse *et al.* 2011). Indeed, limitations in long-established and traditional approaches to health education (St Leger and Nutbeam 2000; Lee *et al.* 2003), to supporting young people's health and wellbeing (Armour *et al.* 2017), and in the pedagogy traditionally applied to teaching about health within physical education, have been acknowledged (Armour and Harris 2013; Haerens *et al.* 2011). In addition, criticisms have been levelled at the simplistic and narrow way in which schools and teachers often engage with health issues (e.g. Evans 2007; Evans *et al.* 2008; Wright and Dean 2007). For example, in their delivery of health, teachers have been found to focus predominantly on instrumental outcomes such as those relating to safety and exercise effects rather than those linked with health benefits and activity promotion (Alfrey and Gard 2014; Harris 2010). Evidently, social media provides another platform for potentially the same simplistic and narrow approach to be reinforced and perpetuated. Further, the ease with which this can occur is apparent in the case studies, for instance, through a limited focus on body transformation videos and information available on YouTube (Chapter 3) or on body image and health shortcuts (Chapter 6).

More fundamentally, though, are concerns regarding the health and obesity discourses which pervade schools (e.g. Evans 2007; Evans *et al.* 2008; Evans and Rich 2011; Gard and Wright 2005; Wright and Dean 2007) and undoubtedly other sites. It is suggested these discourses bear features of and promote a 'performative' culture celebrating comparison, measurement, assessment, and accountability and focus attention on 'corporeal perfection' (e.g. the 'slender ideal') and 'body perfection codes' (defining what and how the body ought to be) (Evans 2007). The concern here is how this performative culture and discourse are then expressed in health-related curricula, pedagogies, and on social media sites and subsequently translated and interpreted by practitioners and young people. Again, it is argued that this tends to be simplistically and narrowly, for example, focusing on body shape, weight, and how the body looks, in turn promoting and potentially leading to harmful thinking, practices, and behaviours (Evans *et al.* 2008; Wright and Dean 2007). The prevalence of these codes within the case studies and the associated dangers were recognised in earlier chapters (Chapters 8, 11, and 12). Examples include the seemingly 'unhealthy' interest shown by some young people in working on the body and body transformation (Chapter 3), and in posting body images (Chapters 4 and 6) and polished and perfect images on Instagram (Chapter 6). Following on from this, given that many adults are uncertain about how to support young people's engagement with social media generally (Shaw *et al.* 2015), and that social media serves to heighten issues surrounding physical activity and health, it seems feasible to conclude that practitioners will equally, if not more so, struggle to deliver health education in the more complex digital media context. Chapter 9 similarly acknowledges this as a challenge for physical education teachers.

In recognition of concerns over the delivery of health and related discourses, calls have been made for a more socially critical perspective to teaching and learning about health and to health knowledge and information (Burrows, Wright, and McCormack 2009; Haerens *et al.* 2011; Quennerstedt 2008). As is apparent from Chapters 8 and 15, some countries, and notably Australia, seem to have made better progress and to be ahead of the game in this regard. Within the Australian curriculum, developing students' 'ability to selectively access and critically analyse information, and take action to promote their own and others' good health' is an explicit and firmly embedded aspect of health and physical education (ACARA 2012, p. 24). Clearly though, supporting young people to develop this ability demands teachers to not only have adequate knowledge and skills but also recognise the need and have the desire to do so.

Evidence however, suggests this may be a challenge. Teachers' lack of a critical approach to health and their uncritical reliance and acceptance of health information from different sources have been reported elsewhere, both generally (Alfrey, Cale, and Webb 2012; Cale, Harris, and Duncombe 2016), and with respect to digital technologies (Casey, Goodyear, and Armour 2017). Casey and colleagues' (2017) pedagogical cases on digital technologies and learning in physical education found little evidence of practitioners' desire to critically evaluate the physical activity and health information they accessed via such means or to explore potentially negative messages with students. As Chapter 1 highlights, if teachers are uncritical and uncertain themselves, this leaves them (and all adults) ill-equipped to protect young people from the negative influences and to optimise the potential of social media with regards health. In line with others' recommendations concerning digital technologies or other media sources (Alfrey, Cale, and Webb 2012; Casey, Goodyear, and Armour 2017; Oliver and Kirk 2016), there is thus a clear need to focus on adults' critical pedagogical response both to health and health-related social media. In short and from an educational point of view, we need to develop critically aware pedagogues (Casey, Goodyear, and Armour 2017) who can support and develop critically aware youngsters.

Another challenge of relevance to social media and health relates to the reported lack of revolution in education (Casey, Goodyear, and Armour 2017). In their research, Casey *et al.* (2017) noted how even among the practitioners who embraced digital technologies, traditional physical education practice remained largely intact, with the technology simply serving to reinforce this. It can therefore be assumed that the same will apply to social media technology and health. Indeed, Chapter 15 cites research which suggests that, as in other areas, digital technologies will be used in health and physical education to deliver more of the same and claims there to be a 'gulf' between the transformative potential of technology and its translation into the classroom. As acknowledged in Chapter 9, these findings reinforce the reputation the physical education profession has for being resistant to change (Alfrey and Gard 2014; Kirk 2010), with teacher-led approaches continuing to dominate practice (Kirk, 2010). With reference to health specifically, Alfrey and Gard (2014, p. 4) refer to the profession as one which is 'steadfastly resistant to change away from the dualistic and instrumental understandings of health and the body ...', towards more 'progressive and student-centred practices and pedagogies'.

What is needed and arguably being called for either implicitly or explicitly throughout this book (e.g. Chapters 8, 9, 12, and 15) is good pedagogical practice with respect to social media, physical activity, and health. Yet, as already alluded to, there are limitations in the existing pedagogies applied to health, and further knowledge about effective health pedagogies is seen as a significant gap in the field (Armour and Harris 2013; Haerens *et al.* 2011; Hodges *et al.* 2017). That said, if we reflect on effective pedagogy generally and consider it in the context of health, and social media and health, there are clear parallels and some key principles and features which should inform our practice. Akin to constructivist learning theories, effective pedagogy and equally effective digital health pedagogy should, I argue, be student-centred, inclusive, contextually relevant, and an active and engaging process. In this context, the desired outcomes should surely be young people who are confident, empowered, independent, and resilient and who value, enjoy, are motivated, and have positive attitudes towards and a desire to lead a healthy, active lifestyle. Earlier authors (Chapters 9 and 12) similarly acknowledge the importance of the latter, affective domain, with Chapter 9 advocating the need for new pedagogies and strategies focusing on this domain specifically. In addition, the opportunities and features of social media (e.g. it is self-directed, and an accessible and active space) lend themselves well to a constructivist approach meaning that, if effective, these positive outcomes should be achievable. Sadly, the evidence from the case studies suggests that social media is failing to promote these outcomes in some young people and, to the contrary, highlights how exclusive and disempowering it can be. Good examples are the behaviours, concerns, and anxieties invoked in the young people over body image posts (Chapter 4) and peer endorsements through 'likes' (Chapter 5). Thus, it seems more attention needs to be paid to the development of effective health pedagogies (Armour and Harris 2013) and digital health pedagogies, perhaps even more so within the social media context, to support practitioners in developing knowledgeable, confident, motivated, and empowered youngsters who can make critically informed decisions about health information, messages, and about their own health and health behaviours.

A final reflection on 'the present' is that, in efforts to achieve the above, social media should, in many respects, be a dream site for educationalists and health promoters because it can overcome many widely reported barriers. Unlike other typical sites for physical activity and health promotion, for example, social media is already extensively used, is contemporary, socially relevant, and culturally accepted by most young people (Casey, Goodyear, and Armour 2017), and it provides constant, immediate, and effortless 24/7 access for the promotion of health and physical activity information and messages. It also provides an informal and relatively free, and adult free, learning environment, in contrast to the structured learning environment of schools, which many young people see as irrelevant and against which they rebel. It is certainly a far cry from the traditional stuffy classroom, physical education changing room, or cold playing field. Related to this, and key to effective physical activity and health promotion and to designing new and successful interventions, is understanding the target group – in this case young people (Cale and Harris 2009; Leahy *et al.* 2016; Oliver and Kirk 2016). In particular, this involves understanding their development, characteristics, preferences, perspectives, and lifestyles (Cale and Harris 2009). Again, social media and social media use are most compatible with these. In short, social media suits young people and reflects them and the way they choose to live their lives, thereby illustrating its enormous potential as a health and health-related learning tool.

The future

Chapter 16 provides a clear steer for the future, summarising the evidence presented in the earlier chapters and presenting new directions for research, policy, and practice relating to young people, social media, physical activity, and health. Specifically, guidance is provided based on the evidence from young people, key stakeholders, and different academic disciplines to support researchers, policy makers, and health and education practitioners/professionals in optimising the potential acknowledged above, as well as mitigating against the risks. The authors also question whether the book has served its purpose and will be 'useful'. In response, I suggest: absolutely. Below, I consider just some of the findings, issues, and guidance outlined in this penultimate chapter and offer some thoughts and suggestions, as appropriate, to trigger further ideas, debate, and developments.

Very apparent in the findings and guidance is the need to engage all health and wellbeing stakeholders across multiple contexts and levels. The importance of a joined-up and consistent approach and messaging is evident if we are to successfully support young people in their engagement with health-related digital media. At the same time, Chapter 16 acknowledges the challenge of identifying messages most relevant to different stakeholder groups and in developing audience-specific messages. Alongside translation of the current guidance and messages, generating more tailored yet still consistent messaging perhaps ought to be the next stage in the research process. This could be achieved most effectively through a process of co-construction or co-refinement with all stakeholders.

Recognising young people's existing critical and other skills and realising the opportunities and the positive health impacts from social media are strongly advocated in Chapter 16 and, as noted earlier, seems a constructive way forward.

Whilst there is consensus among all authors that risk cannot be ignored, over-emphasising risk can be perceived as 'nannying', an approach which is known to be largely ineffective in physical activity and health promotion (Cale and Harris 2009). On the other hand, focusing on 'do' and 'can' messages is empowering and in keeping with the principles of good and effective pedagogy highlighted earlier. It was also very clear in the case studies that over-emphasis on risks, regulatory advice, and an overly protection-oriented approach was not well received by the young people and, indeed, was viewed as unhelpful, irrelevant, frustrating, and even a 'running joke' (Chapter 7).

To facilitate a positive approach and outcomes, Chapter 16 proposes guide-lines and resources to be produced for service providers, schools, teachers, and parents/carers. These outline how young people could be supported, and funds allocated to support professional learning about social media. For these guide-lines to be adopted and ultimately have impact, it seems imperative that they also include strategies and ideas (which could be in the form of tried and tested case studies) on how to integrate the guidelines and resources into different set-tings, whether this be the curriculum, home, community, or other sites. Any support furthermore, I suggest, needs to be mindful of the other competing demands and pressures faced by the adults involved. As noted earlier, with respect primarily to health, these other factors often mean many practitioners fail to engage with relevant professional development, lack adequate knowledge and skills, and/or afford the area relatively limited status and attention.

In addition, if we are to achieve positive outcomes and in turn tackle undesir-able learning outcomes associated with social media engagement, particularly in the school context, then I recommend we establish some consensus and expecta-tions concerning these. These would typically include the knowledge, under-standing, and skills young people require, as well as an understanding of how these can or are likely to be demonstrated in practice. The lack of clarity con-cerning the nature of health knowledge in health and physical education (Armour and Harris 2013) and the health knowledge and experiences young people require to lead healthy, active lifestyles has been acknowledged elsewhere (Cale and Harris 2018). Indeed, in recognition of this some time ago, an 'expert' working group was convened, a key output from which was the publication of national guidance and a set of health-related learning outcomes for young people aged 5–16 years (see Harris 2000; Harris and Cale 2018). Whilst these are com-prehensive in scope in that they incorporate cognitive, affective, and behavioural outcomes, it seems timely now to revisit and extend these to include outcomes relating to digital health. We therefore need to ask and establish what positive health-related social media learning outcomes are important for young people. In other words, what is a health-related social media literate young person? What knowledge, understanding, skills, and attributes are relevant and what does such an individual have/need? Having identified the outcomes, consideration then needs to be paid to how they might be developed, which would ideally entail designing and sharing some evidenced-based, tried and tested strategies and learning activities to support young people in meeting them.

Another key element of the guidance and which is reinforced readily throughout the book is the central involvement of young people (Chapters 8, 9, 10, 14, and 15), something which again is fundamental to developing and delivering good and effective pedagogy. If we are ever to make real headway in supporting, developing, and enhancing young people's health-related knowledge and behaviours then they and their experiences must be at the heart of the process. For too long in research, education, and health, we have worked 'on' rather than 'with' young people, thinking adults 'know best' (Chapter 14). On this, Chapter 14 suggests that, despite being 'trailblazers' in social spaces, young people are deliberately excluded from decision-making which seems ludicrous as well as ethically questionable. As seen in the case studies (Chapters 2–7), young people should not be underestimated and, in fact, are a rich resource upon which to draw. In these chapters, the young people showed maturity and insight in their dialogues, revealing themselves to be reflective, critical, and balanced in many ways. For example, whilst admittedly being confused at times, the young people were nonetheless often questioning or sceptical of health products such as FitTea (Chapter 2), 'waist trainers' (Chapter 6) and/or 'shortcuts' to health (Chapter 6). As recommended in Chapter 16, young people can be actively involved in many ways, including in designing or co-designing initiatives, support, practices, and policies. We therefore need to establish effective ways of working with young people on such developments and recognise their expertise, capacity, and agency. Their continued involvement in research and the student-driven, participatory pedagogies and activist and other approaches highlighted in this book (Chapters 8, 9, and 15) offer much promise in this regard.

On the topic of research, this book makes a significant and much needed contribution to our knowledge and understanding of young people, social media, physical activity, and health, presenting new findings, insights, and a new approach to guide future research. Yet, there are still many gaps in our knowledge. This area and the framework applied in this research are still in their infancy and many questions remain. The authors identify a few pressing areas for attention in Chapter 16 with which I concur. Alongside these, key areas of interest and concern to myself as a researcher and educationalist include social media, diversity and inclusion, and understanding social media use, and experiences of young people of different abilities, disabilities, and learning needs. Indeed, Chapters 11 and 15 raise issues relating to social media and equity, diversity and democracy which are clearly complex and cannot be ignored. As recognised in these earlier chapters, some groups of young people are likely to be more excluded, marginalised, and/or more vulnerable and potentially at risk from social media than others. From the case studies presented here it is also easy to see how social media may contribute to positive outcomes for the confident and clever child, but to negative outcomes for others. Given this, a further interest lies in ultimately establishing and advancing knowledge of effective digital health pedagogies which will enable *all* young people to realise positive health outcomes from social media. This will clearly need to draw on the firm foundations laid by this and the future research proposed in this book.

A further and crucial matter now is knowledge translation, with Chapter 16 pointing to the need for further work and offering suggestions regarding this. Whilst there is evidently much to do to achieve the authors' knowledge translation ambitions, it will be exciting to see this work develop. Certainly, the central involvement of young people, stakeholders, and the collaborative, iterative, and dynamic approach taken through the pedagogical cases model to translate the work and to bridge the gap between theory, research, and practice provide real scope for impact. The output, a valuable, relevant, and thought-provoking professional development learning resource and tool to support and develop adults' practice, represents a significant step. As Chapter 16 highlights, moving forwards, engaging and influencing relevant adults, and monitoring the impact of this is essential.

Concluding remarks

The work presented in this book presents renewed hope and new and exciting opportunities to positively impact the health and lives of young people. The evidence and analysis presented in this chapter, however, suggests that first, many adults, including teachers, need to address a number of issues and their own shortcomings with regards to young people, social media, physical activity, and health. Noteworthy though, is that many of these issues are not new but are long-standing within the field of physical activity and health more broadly. Thus, at present, we seem to have a case of 'new media, same old issues'. Yet, adding social media to the mix represents a powerful triplex and offers new possibilities. Addressing current challenges and shortcomings will require honest reflection, recognition of a professional and collective responsibility for the health and wellbeing of our youth, and a firm commitment to one's own as well as young people's development in this regard. Only in this way will we be able to seize the opportunities afforded by social media to support, empower, and protect young people with respect to their health, health behaviours, and engagement with health information and messages. In addition, regardless of context and given that all sites are learning spaces, I advocate that our collective efforts need to be underpinned by good pedagogical principles and practice. Finally, to generate further debate, discussion, and facilitate professional learning, Chapter 16 concludes by encouraging us all to digitally engage with the authors about this research. This engagement is clearly to be welcomed and 'healthy', and I look forward to doing so and to further developments.

References

Alfrey, L. and Gard, M., 2014. A crack where the light gets in: A study of health and physical education teachers' perspectives on fitness testing as a context for learning about health. *Asia-Pacific Journal of Health, Sport and Physical Education*, 5(1), 3–18.

Alfrey, L., Cale, L., and Webb L., 2012. Physical education teachers' continuing professional development in health related exercise. *Physical Education and Sport Pedagogy*, 17(5), 477–491.

Armour, K.M. and Harris, J., 2013. Making the case for developing new PE-for-health pedagogies. *Quest*, 65(2), 201–219.

Armour, K.M., Quennerstedt, M., Chambers, F., and Makopoulou, K., 2017. What is 'effective' CPD for contemporary physical education teachers? A Deweyan framework. *Sport, Education and Society*, 22(7), 799–811.

Australian Curriculum, Assessment and Reporting Authority ACARA., 2012. *The Health and Physical Education Curriculum F-10*. Sydney: ACARA.

Brusseau, T., Kulinna, P., and Cothran, D., 2011. Health and physical activity content knowledge of Pima children. *The Physical Educator*, 68(2), 66–77.

Burrows, L., 2008. 'Fit, fast, and skinny': New Zealand school students 'talk' about health. *Journal of Physical Education New Zealand*, 41(3), 26–36.

Burrows, L., 2010. Kiwi kids are Weet-Bix™ kids – body matters in childhood. *Sport, Education and Society*, 15(2), 235–251.

Burrows, L. and Wright, J., 2010. The good life: New Zealand children's perspectives on health and self. *Sport, Education and Society*, 9(2), 193–205.

Burrows, L. and McCormack, J., 2014. Doing it for themselves: A qualitative study of children's engagement with public health agendas in New Zealand. *Critical Public Health*, 24(2), 159–170.

Burrows, L., Wright, J., and McCormack, J., 2009. Dosing up on food and physical activity: New Zealand children's ideas about 'health'. *Health Education Journal*, 68(3), 157–169.

Cale, L. and Harris, J., 2009. *Getting the Buggers Fit (second edition)*. London: Continuum.

Cale, L. and Harris, J., 2018. The role of knowledge and understanding in fostering physical literacy. *Journal of Teaching in Physical Education*, 37(3), 280–287.

Cale, L., Harris, J., and Duncombe, R., 2016. Promoting physical activity in secondary schools. Growing expectations: Same old issues. *European Physical Education Review*, 22(4), 526–544.

Cardon, G.M., Van Acker, R., Seghers, J., Martelaer, K., and Haerens, L.L., 2012. Physical activity promotion in schools: Which strategies do schools (not) implement and which socioecological factors are associated with implementation? *Health Education Research*, 27(3), 470–483.

Casey, A., Goodyear, V.A., and Armour, K.M., 2017. Rethinking the relationship between pedagogy, technology and learning in health and physical education. *Sport, Education and Society*, iFirst Article.

Castelli, D. and Williams, L., 2007. Health-related fitness and physical education teachers' content knowledge. *Journal of Teaching in Physical Education*, 26(1), 3–19.

Evans, J., 2007. Health education or weight management in schools? *Cardiometabolic Risk and Weight Management*, 2(2), 12–16.

Evans, J., Rich, E., Davies, B., and Allwood, R., 2008. *Education, Disordered Eating and Obesity Discourse. Fat Fabrications*. Routledge: Oxon.

Evans, J. and Rich, E., 2011. Body policies and body pedagogies; every child matters in totally pedagised schools. *Journal of Education Policy*, 26(2), 311–329.

Gard, M. and Wright, J., 2005. *The Obesity Epidemic: Science, Ideology and Morality*. London: Routledge.

Haerens, L., Kirk, D., Cardon, G., and De Bourdeaudhuij, I., 2011. Toward the development of a pedagogical model for health-based physical education. *Quest*, 63, 321–338.

Harris, J., 2000. *Health-related Exercise in the National Curriculum*. Leeds, UK: Human Kinetics.

Harris, J., 2010. Health-related physical education. *In:* R. Bailey, ed., *Physical Education for Learning: A Guide for Secondary Schools*. London: Continuum, 26–36.

Harris, J. and Cale, L., 2018. *Promoting Active Lifestyles in Schools*. Leeds: Human Kinetics.

Harris, J. and Leggett, G., 2015. Influences on the expression of health within physical education curricula in secondary schools in England and Wales. *Sport Education and Society*, 20(7), 908–923.

Harris, J., Cale, L., Duncombe, R., and Musson, H., 2018. Young people's knowledge and understanding of health, fitness and physical activity: Issues, divides and dilemmas. *Sport, Education and Society*, 23(5), 407–420.

Hastie, P., 2017. Revisiting the national physical education content standards: What do we really know about our achievement of the physically educated/literate person? *Journal of Teaching in Physical Education*, 36, 3–19.

Hodges, M., Kulinna, P.M., Lee, C., and Kwon, J.Y., 2017. Professional development and teacher perceptions of experiences teaching health-related fitness knowledge. *Journal of Teaching in Physical Education*, 36, 32–39.

Hooper, O., 2018. *Health(y) Talk: Pupil's Conceptions of Health within Physical Education*. Doctoral Thesis: Loughborough University.

Jourdan, D., McNamara, P.M., Simar, C., Geary, T., and Pommier, J., 2010. Factors influencing the contribution of staff to health education in schools. *Health Education Research*, 25(4), 519–530.

Keating, X.D. Harrison, L., Chen, L., Xiang, P., Lambdin, D., Dauenhauer, D., Rotich, W., and Pinero, J.C., 2009. An analysis of research on student health-related fitness knowledge in K-16 physical education programs. *Journal of Teaching in Physical Education*, 28, 333–349.

Kirk, D., 2010. *Physical Education Futures*. Oxon: Routledge.

Kulinna, H., McCaughtry, N., Martin, J.J., Cothran, D., and Faust, R., 2008. The influence of professional development on teachers' psychosocial perceptions of teaching a health-related physical education curriculum. *Journal of Teaching in Physical Education* 27, 292–307.

Larsen, T., Tjomsland, H., and Samdal, O., 2013. Physical activity in schools. A qualitative case study of eight Norwegian schools' experiences with the implementation of a national policy. *Health Education*, 113(1), 52–63.

Leahy, D., Burrows, L., McCuaig, L., Wright, J., and Penney, D., 2016. *School Health Education in Changing Times*. London: Routledge.

Lee A., Tsang C., Lee, S.H., and To, C.Y., 2003. A comprehensive 'Healthy Schools Programme' to promote school health: The Hong Kong experience in joining the efforts of health and education sectors. *Journal of Epidemiology and Community Health*, 57, 174–177.

Marks, R., 2008. Schools and health education. What works, what is needed, and why? *Health Education*, 109(1), 4–8.

McMullen, J., Chroinin, D., Pogorzelska, M., and van der Mars, H., 2015. International approaches to whole-of-school physical activity promotion. *Quest* 67, 384–399.

Oliver, K.M. and Kirk, D., 2016. Towards an activist approach to research and advocacy for girls and physical education. *Physical Education and Sport Pedagogy*, 21, 313–327.

Powell, D. and Fitzpatrick, K., 2015. 'Getting fit basically just means, like, nonfat': children's lessons in fitness and fatness. *Sport, Education and Society*, 20, 4, 463–484.

Puhse, U., Barker, D., Brettschneider, W.D., Feldmeth, A.K., Anne, K., Gerlach, E., McCuaig, L., McKenzie, T.L., and Gerber, M., 2011. International approaches to health-oriented physical education: Local health debates and differing conceptions of health. *International Journal of Physical Education*, 3, 2–15.

Quennerstedt, M., 2008. Exploring the relation between physical activity and health – a salutogenic approach to physical education. *Sport, Education and Society*, 13(3), 276–283.

Roth, M. and Stamatakis, E., 2010. Linking young people's knowledge of public health guidelines to physical activity levels in England. *Pediatric Exercise Science*, 22, 467–476.

Shaw, J.M., Mitchell, C.A., Welch, A.J., and Williamson, M.J., 2015. Social media used as a health intervention in adolescent health: A systematic review of the literature. *Digital Health*, 1, 1–10.

Speller, V., Byrne, J., Dewhirst S., Almond, P., Mohebati, L., Norman, M., Polack, S., Memon, A., Grace, M., Margetts, B., and Roderick, P., 2010. Developing trainee school teachers' expertise as health promoters. *Health Education*, 110(6), 490–507.

St Leger, L. and Nutbeam, D., 2000. Research into health promoting schools. *Journal of School Health*, 70(5), 257–259.

Wright, J. and Dean, R., 2007. A balancing act. Problematising prescriptions about food and weight in school health texts. *Journal of Didactics and Educational Policy*, 16(2), 75–94.

Index

Page numbers in bold denote tables, those in italics denote figures.

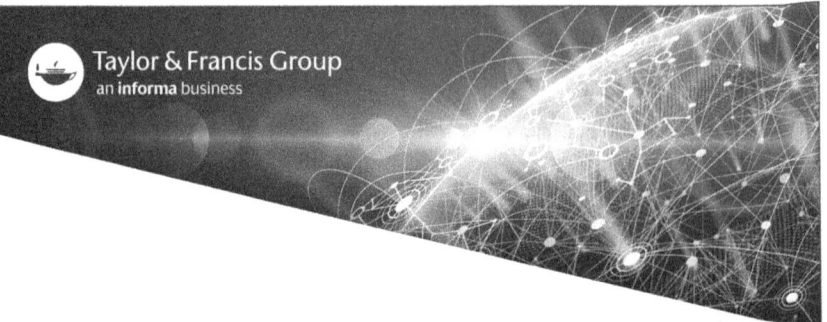
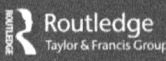
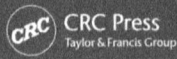